HOW TO TAKE CHARGE OF YOUR CHILD'S EARLY EDUCATION

J. Robert Parkinson

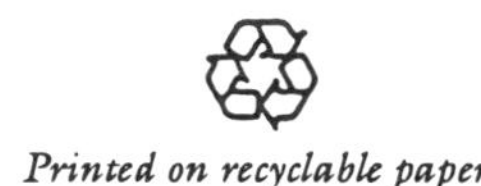

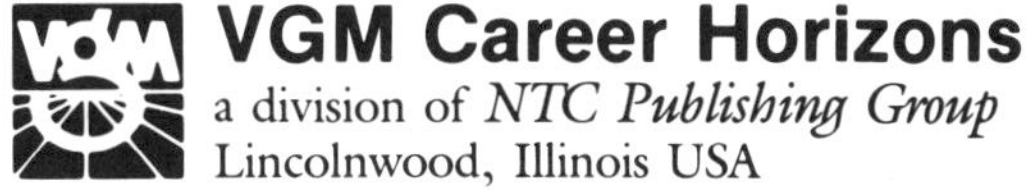

VGM Career Horizons
a division of *NTC Publishing Group*
Lincolnwood, Illinois USA

Library of Congress Cataloging-in-Publication Data

Parkinson, J. Robert (John Robert)
    How to take charge of your child's early education / J. Robert
Parkinson.
        p.   cm.
    Includes bibliographical references.
    ISBN 0-8442-4394-9
    1. Early childhood education—Parent participation.   2. School
choice.   I. Title.
LB1139.35.P37P27   1996
372.2—dc20   95–30146
                                                                                    CIP

Published by VGM Career Horizons, a division of NTC Publishing Group
4255 West Touhy Avenue
Lincolnwood (Chicago), Illinois 60646-1975, U.S.A.

5 6 7 8 9 0 VP 9 8 7 6 5 4 3 2 1

Contents

About the Author

J. Robert Parkinson is presently an associate professor at Northwestern University. He has been a teacher, principal, and central office administrator. He has served as an educational consultant to numerous organizations and institutions. He was formerly Dean of the Institute of Research at the National College of Education, Director of Educational Research for Bell and Howell, and is the author of numerous articles on education.

Dr. Parkinson is also the host of the award-winning weekly radio program "For Your Consideration." With his wife, Eileen, he writes, produces, and hosts television documentaries under the company banner EIROPA Communications Group.

Foreword

This book is a timely, informative, and important guide for today's parents. At a time when change is occurring at an astounding rate and education is seemingly more important than ever, parents frequently are bewildered as to what the future holds for them and especially their children. It is increasingly difficult for parents to decide on what manner of education will most successfully prepare their children for a world that they cannot predict. In addition, the critical focus on schooling at the national, state, and local levels contributes to parents' sense of uneasiness and concern that they must do everything necessary to assure their children successful learning experiences throughout the school-age years.

Dr. Parkinson has succeeded in providing the needed advice to parents for the role that begins in the home and extends into the school years. His emphasis on the family as the first educator affirms the parents' importance to their young children. He reflects the wisdom of philosophers of past ages as he offers encouraging suggestions to parents in recognizing their importance in the educations of their children. He describes the role played by their own attitudes toward learning in providing children with the desire to know about and understand themselves and the world around them.

Advice on selection of toys, household materials, and experiences that contribute to children's development of social, intellectual, affective, and physical abilities is provided in a clear manner throughout the book. He provides useful information regarding the criteria in determining whether a personal computer will be appropriate to specific learning needs and offers sources to gain further information regarding computers and computer-assisted learning.

Throughout the chapters regarding selection of schools, Dr. Parkinson emphasizes two important points: partnership and participation. He carefully points to facts that indicate that parental involvement in selecting good schools as well as a commitment to continued participation in the educational life and goals of the schools, are critical to sustaining the academic achievement of their children. Criteria and questions relating to the professional abilities of teachers, principals, librarians, and other staff who assist in children's educational life, is provided. Parents are encouraged to be as knowledgeable as possible in relation to the formal aspects of schooling.

The greatest impression that parents will have in reading this book is that their child's education—the development of mind, skill, character, and knowledge is a process that is best begun within the home and is best promoted with the full participation, knowledge, and commitment of the family. Dr. Parkinson provides parents with knowledge of the basic foundations that they can provide that ensure the best possible education for their children: appropriate home-learning activities; role modelling for a continued interest in learning; selection of high-quality educational institutions and professional staff; and methods of integrating the home and school in their childrens' education through initiating and maintaining positive parent-teacher relationships.

As the first century philosopher, Quintilianus said, "I would have [parents] conceive the highest hope for their [child] from the moment of birth. If so, they will never be more careful about the groundwork of their [child's] education." (Ulich, 1954, *Three Thousand Years of Educational Wisdom,* p. 103)

Dr. Parkinson's book provides the twentieth-century parent with the blueprints for beginning to lay such a groundwork.

Susan Belgrad
Professor of Early Childhood Education
National College of Education

Dedication

To my wife, Eileen, for the encouragement to write this book, and to each young child whose education may be affected by it.

Construct a Plan 1

If you don't know where you want to go you won't know when you get there.

The title of this book was chosen carefully to place the responsibility exactly where it belongs—on you. As a parent, it's your job to assure your child receives the education to which he or she is entitled. Many times parents think the school is the responsible party. WRONG!

The school has a function, but the school's agenda in this situation is very different from yours. Your agenda is to focus on *your* child. The school's agenda is to provide as much as they can for every child that attends. That— in just terms of numbers—is very different. No one cares as much for your child as you do. No one knows as much about your child as you. So you must take charge if you want the job of education done right.

That doesn't mean you can or should do it alone. You need the school to play its part, but that's just what it is—a part. You have to take major responsibility, or it won't get done the way you want.

But "taking charge" means you must *know* about it.

You must know what schools, teachers, and principals can do. You must know something about curriculum—about the law. And, you must know something about evaluation: of the school, the people who work there, and the materials that are used.

Teachers are in the evaluation business—they evaluate your child every day. Often, however, they don't like to be the ones being evaluated. You just have to be ready for some defensiveness. But don't ever hesitate to evaluate them—just be sure you evaluate the right things! That's one of the items we'll cover in this book.

What Do You Want?

One of the major difficulties, however, is what should you look for? You must be very clear about *what you want.* However, be careful. Many of us are tempted to think schools today should be like they were years ago—when we went to school. We often hear "This is what we did when I went to school, and look at me now. It was good for me, so it's good for my child." That might not be so.

What worked for us when we were children was part of *that* world, that time. The world today is different, and the school experience might have to be different too. So use caution when taking charge. "Different" by itself doesn't make anything better or worse. Decide what you want for your child, and then try this: Write it down on a piece of paper. Be very specific about what you want.

This sounds easy, but you'll probably find it difficult when you face that blank piece of paper. The words might not come out easily. This happens because we often "fool" ourselves when we just *think* about something. If we have to face the discipline of the blank page we really do have to know. If we don't know, we won't be able to write it. If we can't write it we probably won't get it because we don't know what "it" is! If we don't know what "it" is how are we ever going to tell someone else—or how will we know if we ever do get "it?"

So before you begin your exploration—your evaluation—write down what you want for your child.

Be Specific

This is one of the areas where you, as a parent, and school organizations will differ. Schools often deal in general statements and labels like "making progress," "works cooperatively," "being a good citizen," "showing growth," etc. How can you measure those?

You want specifics like "can count to ___," "can write his or her name," "can spell the name of the school, the teacher, the street," "can solve quadratic equations"—well maybe not that one—at least not yet.

The point is simple. If you can be specific you can observe and measure. If you are vague so will your outcomes be vague. That won't help your young child.

Certainly this will be a difficult task, but raising a child *is* a difficult task. Being specific will help. You don't have time for "trial and error." The clock keeps on running. If there is a mistake you can't go back and start over; you have to continue from that point. Time has been lost, and you can't get it back. You must be right the first time. Someone once said "life isn't a dress rehearsal." That's correct. You get one try. If you miss the first time you have to press onward—you can't hit your internal "rewind" button and simply repeat.

So focus. That will help you talk to the teachers and to ask good questions. Good questions require good, focused answers. That's what you want from your child's teacher!

And that's *your* responsibility. To "take charge" means "to know." Only you know what you want. So tell the teachers.

A Partnership

There is another factor we must discuss here. So far, the emphasis has been on you deciding what you want for your young child. But this shouldn't be construed to mean that only you will have all the answers. The teachers and other education professionals have a very important role to play. They are the experts in the "how" part. You focus on "what," and they concentrate on "how." A great partnership!

That's what the education process is—a partnership. You, your child, the teachers, and everyone in his/her life contributes to the total education. Remember school is a part of the child's education. That one person, your child, will interact with many "teachers" and situations, and they all add up to the total outcome.

As we go through this book and suggest over and over that you "ask questions," "evaluate," "demand answers," etc., the emphasis isn't on a competition. The emphasis is one of equal talking to equal. Your relationship with your young child's school should not be adversarial, but it must be focused, and you must set that focus. You must be certain that whatever happens, happens *on purpose* and not by accident.

All of us do many things by habit; we don't always make conscious decisions about everything. It is only when we question our own behavior that we make changes. So it is with teachers and schools. Things get done by habit—not necessarily by design. Education is not a "one size fits all" situation.

Since your child is unique (maybe not quite as unique as you might think, though) so must the education experience be unique. It must be tailor made. Of course, some selected pieces will fit most of the subjects, but the overall fit isn't mass production.

Allow me to draw an analogy about this "partnership" between parent and school—about the "what" and the "how" of the education experience.

It is very much like taking a road trip in your car. Before you start out you decide where you want to go. Once that decision is made you can start off with a purpose—the destination. This is the "what," the outcome.

You are free to select the route you will take to get to that destination. It might be the "fastest" or the "scenic" or the "necessary" one because of road construction. But whichever one you select, you will get to the destination. The route in the analogy is the "how."

Clearly, you need both a "what" and a "how." If you don't know where you want to go, it doesn't make any difference which way you go. True, you might end up in a nice place, but that's risky. So you plan, and then you execute that plan.

In education for your young child, you decide *what* you want and the teachers concentrate on the *how* to get there. But the "what" must come first!

As with the road trip, without a plan you *might* end up in a nice place. In your child's education, without a plan the education *might* be good, but do you want to take that chance? Or to put this another way: If you take the time to plan a road trip doesn't it make sense to plan your young child's education? Doesn't it make sense to "take charge?"

Of course it does! So get started. It's your job, your responsibility. The final outcome will be your reward. Your child *will* get to that "nice place," and you'll help him/her get there on purpose!

So, let's begin!

A Beginning

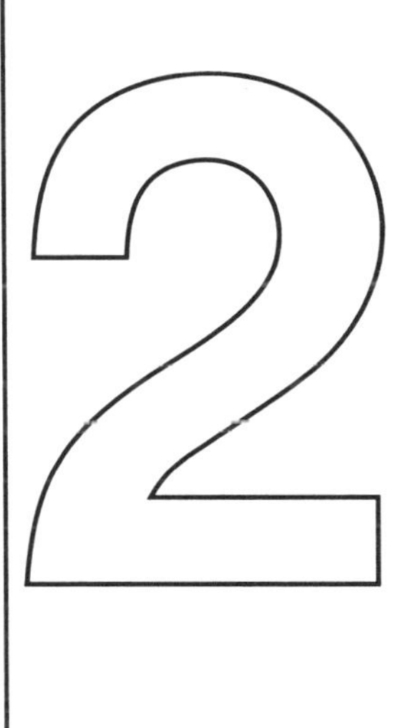

Parents throughout the country share many common experiences. One of those experiences lasts a long time: it can provide great joy, great reward, and sometimes great disappointment and frustration.

That common experience revolves around observing their children learn—at home, then in the neighborhood, and finally at school.

The learning that takes place at home is easily observed. It is usually under reasonable control, and it is usually productive. Children learn to walk, talk, feed themselves, play games, get along with siblings and parents; and they master a host of other skills.

In the neighborhood they learn to get along with other children, share toys, learn the rules of games, and travel to their "special places."

Parents seem to have little difficulty in dealing with how their children learn things at home and in the neighborhood, but when the children reach school age a variety of problems develop.

Parents are faced with difficult questions that they can't answer without help.

- What school should my children attend?
- What kind of teachers will they have?
- What kind of work will they do?
- What will they learn?
- How can I be sure of the steps to take?

Every parent asks these questions in one way or another and experiences the same anxieties about how the next generation will be prepared for adulthood. Of course, parents usually don't think in such general terms, but rather in terms of "What will school mean for *my* child?" And that's how it should be.

Often, the anxiety that parents feel stems from not knowing as much about "the system" as they would like, not knowing what specific questions to ask, what options are available, where to seek assistance, and how to take appropriate action where it is needed. This book is designed to do three things:

- Raise questions.
- Suggest some answers.
- Recommend further action the reader can take.

This book is intended, further, to address current issues and concerns about education and schools and to identify areas that could become concerns in the not-to-distant future.

Two specific recommendations can be made immediately.

- Never hesitate to ask questions about your children's school, their teachers, their experiences, and their activities.

- Don't wait to see if everything will turn out OK. You don't have time for that—and neither does your child.

A Sense of Urgency

To give emphasis to the need for a strong *sense of urgency* about your child's education, as well as the education of all children, consider the following situation.

Imagine for a moment that you are standing on a riverbank looking at the water. Although you are aware of movement, the river looks the same much of the time. What you are viewing, however, is constantly changing. The water in front of you just a moment ago is now moving rapidly downstream. What was upstream is now in front of you—and almost instantly—it's gone. The movement, the replacement, continues.

When we look at schools, they too seem to be what they were for as long as schools have existed. Children and teachers are always there: entering, going to classes, playing, and graduating. But when we look carefully we see that they, like the river, are constantly changing. The littlest ones have grown up, and they will be replaced by others, many of whom have not yet been born.

The school population moves so rapidly that if children miss out on training at a particular point it can only be picked up someplace downstream. It can't simply be inserted in what should have been the original location. You can't turn back time, and supply what is needed as early in the child's life as you might have.

As we think about schools and education we must be filled with a sense of urgency in order to be prepared for the optimum growth our children can achieve at any given age.

We don't have the luxury of endless time—we can't spend years and years contemplating and debating what we want in our young children's educational resources— we must research, evaluate, and make choices early. We can't freeze the moment, until we have leisurely considered all the options, or completed all the research and investigation that we might wish.

Our population keeps changing! In less than five years, the babies being born now will already have completed their preschool education; in only eight years, they will have completed all their primary school years. Children have only one chance at an education: it is necessary for all adults, and especially parents, to be prepared to make sure that one chance pays off.

Preparation, though perhaps complicated at times, is not difficult, and it is certainly not impossible! All of us, in one form or another, have experienced teaching and learning situations at home, in our neighborhoods, and in schools. We rely upon many memories of our own satisfaction and successes in learning situations in teaching our own children; and these memories are valuable. They can't, however, do the whole job. Many of us feel we don't really know what advantages are available today for teaching our children at home. Many of us feel we don't really know what schools are all about today; or what we can do to influence what happens there.

In a time when educational methods and theories are under constant challenge, and changes occur rapidly in even the earliest school situations; when we have available to us many different kinds of child care facilities, thousands of different toys and games of various educational worth, and an increasing population in early childhood and primary grade classrooms, we need to have information and principles upon which we can rely, to make the best possible choices.

The success of our country has been based upon participatory democracy; the success of our children's educations can likewise be based upon participatory parenting and teaching. We can and must participate in our young children's educations, if we want them to acquire and develop the skills needed to participate in their own ways in their future society as effectively as they should.

In the following pages you will find information that will be helpful in making choices to prepare for an optimal educational experience for your young child—at home, in day care and child care facilities, and in primary school situations. It is hoped that these pages will help you understand more of what to expect, what can be done to make the most of learning situations, what cannot be done, and what to do if you encounter problems.

Where Does It Start?

What happens to children once they enter school is, to a large extent, determined by their experiences at home long before that first day.

We've all heard about the amount of time the average child spends in front of a television set. That will be discussed in some detail in another section of this book. What we want to focus on here is the way a child learns about herself or himself and how he or she feels about the learning process in general. Of course, children never think about it that way; but we will.

Take, for example, the idea of self-confidence in decision-making. Obviously, we can't deal with that entire issue here, but for purposes of illustration, let's examine how we can help—or hinder—a child and her or his feelings about making decisions.

Making Decisions

All of us must make decisions throughout our lives, and the comfort and confidence we display are directly related to the early experiences we had as children.

Very often parents unintentionally convince their children that they can't make good decisions. They set up situations and conditions which prove to their children that they are incapable of such tasks.

For example: picture this scene in a local grocery store.

> Father asks son: "What kind of cereal do you want for breakfast?"
> Son answers: "XYZ brand!"
> Father says: "Oh, that's not good for you. It has too much sugar."
> Son: "But I like it."
> Father: "I know, but let's get ABC brand—it's better for you."

Or, imagine a similar situation between a parent and child in a clothing store.

> Mother: "What color dress do you want?"
> Daughter: "Green."
> Mother: "Green doesn't look good on you. Let's get the blue one."

In each case the parent gave the child the opportunity to make a decision, and then told the child the decision was a poor one. With repeated opportunities like these any child would soon learn that he or she really isn't very good at making decisions. Maybe this kind of early learning even happened to us, and now we have difficulty making decisions! The child will hesitate to make up her or his own mind, and he or she will learn to look to others for guidance. As parents we like to offer such guidance, but in later years, and they are not too far away, we will insist that the child "think for herself or himself." We don't want our children just following others and doing "what everyone else is doing."

If young children don't get experience now, how are they going to get good at it? If they are not allowed to try and then assess the results of their choices how can we expect them to take chances and rely on their own thinking? There is no doubt about it, decision making consists of taking chances. The extent of the chance, of course, is directly related to the amount of information that the decision maker has, but it is nevertheless a chance.

Asking Questions

Now the parents in our two scenes are interested in their children. The father doesn't want his son to eat too much sugar, and the mother doesn't want her daughter to look less than her best, but what can they do? They can't let the decisions stand, but could have done something quite different in the first place.

The problem developed because of the way in which the questions were asked.

"What kind . . ." and "What color . . ." are wide open questions. There are no limits to them. The children had unlimited options, and they made their decisions based on their own experiences. The parents, on the other hand, had more and different experience so they made "better" decisions for the children. All the children learned from the exercise, though, was that their decisions were not accepted—even though they were invited to make them. What they learned was not a positive outcome, but a negative one.

The parents could have provided a chance for their children to practice decision making by controlling the situations with better questions. They could easily have limited the choices, based upon their greater knowledge and preference. Limiting choices also makes the task of decision making less frightening for all people, regardless of age.

The father could have asked, "Would you like ABC brand cereal or KLM brand cereal for breakfast?"

The mother could have asked, "Would you prefer the blue dress or the white one?"

In each case the child gets to make the decision, but the parent keeps control right from the start. By offering a better choice, the parent offers a situation in which the child can succeed. It isn't necessary, then, to veto the child's choice. On the contrary, because of the predetermined limitations the parent can reinforce the "excellent" choice the child made. This way no matter which items the children select, they are the right ones. The children feel good. Confidence in their own abilities increases while the parents maintain control and continue to provide effective guidance. This is a win–win situation.

As you take control of your child's education right from those early days, you help her or him to feel good about thinking and decision making by letting her or him make decisions. Remember: *control the situation by limiting the choices to just a few—all of which will be okay.*

Decision making is hard enough under the best of conditions; it shouldn't be made even more difficult with too many options. And once you allow the child to make a decision, you want to be able to allow the decision to stand. If you aren't willing to accept your child's decision, don't set up the conditions that will require one to be made.

Planning

Planning on the part of the parent will go a long way in the life of the young child. That positive experience will be very important in later years when the impact and importance of the decisions are more significant than clothing colors or breakfast cereals.

Similar planning in other learning areas will pay off, too. In the earliest situations of learning play, when your child is still a small baby, you can plan to allow the child to experiment and to learn in controlled situations.

When the child becomes interested in using table utensils, a cup, a bowl, and in feeding others, you can prepare the child's food so that one item can be dealt with at a time. A young baby who can move a spoon into and out of the food dish, and learn to enjoy learning to use the utensil, will be much more confident and satisfied than the baby who has three utensils, a glass, a cup and saucer, a bowl and plate all in place at once. Each item can be introduced, one at a time, as the child becomes accustomed to, and confident in using each one.

At a little later stage, toys can be controlled in a similar way. A play pen or play area that is littered with many toys is more frustrating, less efficient as a learning area, and ultimately even more boring to the child than a play area in which only one or two toys are available until they have been thoroughly explored and experimented with.

Looking ahead a little, controlling the number of options, and providing guidance, will help your child to build confidence, practice motor and observational skills, and learn much more quickly. And your child will develop the ability to deal with the environment and its opportunities.

Learning vs. Teaching

Regardless of how sophisticated society becomes, or how well educated parents are, each child enters the world only with *potential*. There is potential to achieve something, to become something, to acquire something, but that potential must be nurtured if it is to develop.

What is done to, for, and with children will determine to a large extent what they will become as adults. Certainly, there are no guarantees. We know that there are numerous instances where children have succeeded—or failed—in spite of what was done to or provided for them. But we know also that the learning environment has an effect, and usually it is an important one.

This is where the concept of "equality" comes in. The truth of the matter is simply "we are not all equal." Period. Every one of us is unique—different. We are not the same as anyone else. We never were, and we never will be.

Now that doesn't mean "better" or "worse." It just means "different." Those differences, however, must be addressed in every educational setting in which our children find themselves.

The circumstances into which we are born are different than those of anyone else—even our own brothers and sisters. After all, when our older siblings were born into the family we weren't there yet. And for our younger siblings we were there! The time was different; the financial conditions were different; there was a different amount of room in the house or apartment. Everything is different and unique for each one of us.

So it stands to reason that we see our world just a little differently than anyone else sees it. And so, our teachers—both formal and informal—should see and treat each of us just a little differently than they treat anyone else in order to help us learn.

Growth and Development

It is significant to realize that growth and development are very personal and absolutely individualized. Each of us must develop to her or his own potential; no one can do it for us. Others can establish conditions and provide environments and opportunities, but each individual must assimilate all such data in order to make use of it.

In very simple terms, no one can learn anything for us; we must learn for ourselves. Each skill and each bit of knowledge must be acquired. We must all go through the many steps from having nothing at all to achieving what ever level of knowledge is ultimately ours.

As we think about taking charge of our young child's education, we must keep in mind that the emphasis should be on *learning* rather than on *teaching*. This emphasis is usually established at home where even as adults, much of our behavior indicates recognition and support of that process. When a child enters the formal school environment, however, the school system often gives greater emphasis to teaching than to learning. This is not simply playing games with words; rather, there is a great distinction between the two processes.

Let's look at the differences between these two approaches.

If the emphasis in an educational institution is on teaching, then the processes that are used, the materials employed, the schedules built, and the language and techniques applied are all for the benefit and convenience of the institution and those who work within it. The faculty, administration, support personnel, etc., make up the rules and then carry them out. Students have little, if any, opportunity to contribute to this process although they are the reason for the existence of the institution in the first place. Students are expected to adapt and to "fit in." If, on the other hand, the emphasis in an institution is on learning, then the process, materials, schedules, language, techniques, etc., are for the benefit and convenience of the students.

When an educational institution operates with the latter emphasis, the teaching task is much more difficult than when teaching is the primary goal. Because each child is unique and must learn everything for her- or himself, we can see that in a learning focused environment, many opportunities and options must be available in order to provide for the varied learning needs of the total student population.

This difficulty or challenge shouldn't be a surprise to anyone, nor should it upset anyone. After all, it has been pointed out frequently that the schools are for the students, not the teachers. Therefore, the challenges of providing opportunities to benefit each and every student should be expected. If it is true that students must learn for themselves, and no one can learn for them, then we must ask ourselves, what must a student learn? Well, we know there are many specific areas, but for the sake of discussion, let's generalize a bit.

Skills

The first learning task is to *acquire* certain skills, and the second learning task is to *apply* these skills. Clearly, without skills there can be no applications.

What are some of these basic skills? Social interaction, acquiring language, understanding numbers, reading, and writing constitute a few of them.

Extending this thought further, we can reason that after a child learns to read he can appreciate a novel; after he knows how to write, he can produce a short story; after he understands numbers, he can balance a checkbook—well, maybe! None of these tasks can be carried out, however, without first acquiring additional, specific skills. Certainly there are many interrelations of skills and many combinations so we won't attempt to examine all of them here. That's not necessary to make the point that learning is individual, personal, and sequential. Throughout this book our emphasis will be on learning.

The educational process is complex, the education community is large, educational institutions are firmly established, but the basic principle is simple and clear-cut. Because each child must learn everything for himself, by himself, the role of adults is to set up the conditions and options that enable learning to take place. So, let's look at some of the factors related to these conditions and options.

Work and Play

While young children are at home, long before they go to school, they learn many things. We discussed some in the previous section.

The amazing thing is that all the learning is fun. Young children ask questions because they enjoy getting the information. In fact, most children are so eager to collect information that we say they are driving us crazy asking "why?," "when?," "where?," "how?" Most of the time, answering just once enables the children to add the new information to their rapidly growing data banks. Learning in this period is fun, and most children go at it with a vengeance.

Then they go to school.

For too many children learning isn't just fun now—or it isn't supposed to be, anyway. Once in school, learning becomes *work*. There is *seat work, board work,* and *home-work*. Work, work, work has replaced fun, fun, fun. Somehow, young children must come to terms with this situation. They must *work* on all of their subjects or they won't learn. They have already learned a great deal, but until school, they never thought of any of that activity as "work."

Very few adults like to work for the sake of working. Most of us work for a variety of rewards: money, travel, security, creativity, etc. Many people truly like their jobs because of the rewards they receive. This should also be true for children. If they can see rewards they will devote the energy needed to complete an assignment. But they must be able to see those rewards and not have to wait "until they grow up." Such long range goal setting is almost impossible for a child. Deferred gratification is a hard concept to sell to anyone, and it is particularly difficult for a child.

Already in their young lives they have learned and retained words, numbers, and various skills. They did so because the rewards were immediate. The information had immediate value to the young children and they were able to use it well in their daily lives. The name of an object was learned because there was an immediate need for it, not because ". . . it will be good for you when you are an adult."

At various stages, children can learn untold quantities of song lyrics, batting averages, phone numbers, and a host of other things because there is an immediate perceived value. That learning is never thought of as work.

Learning a song lyric is fun, but learning a poem to recite in class is "memorization." Even the word itself sounds intimidating: "Memorization!" Who would want to do something called that, when one can just as easily, simply *learn* something? Fun is always more appealing than work.

If you want to get a feel for what happens when the fun of learning is replaced by the work of schooling, pay a visit to your local elementary school the day school opens in the fall. Look at the "little kids" all happy and eager to get started. Then look at the "big kids." They aren't nearly as excited about going to school as their younger colleagues are.

Now ask yourself a question. What has the school system done to these children? What has happened to change the excited young ones into the bored, complacent older ones?

Has "work" been overused and overemphasized in favor of the fun and excitement of just simply learning? Work is hard. Learning shouldn't be seen as work, but an adventure—as fun. People of any age will expend a great deal of effort in pursuit of enjoyable activities much more willingly than they will in just working.

If adults do that, why should we expect any less from children? After all, they have a lot more energy to use. Why not channel it in a constructive direction? And, to use that phrase again, the results will be "good for them when they grow up!"

What Should I Do at Home?

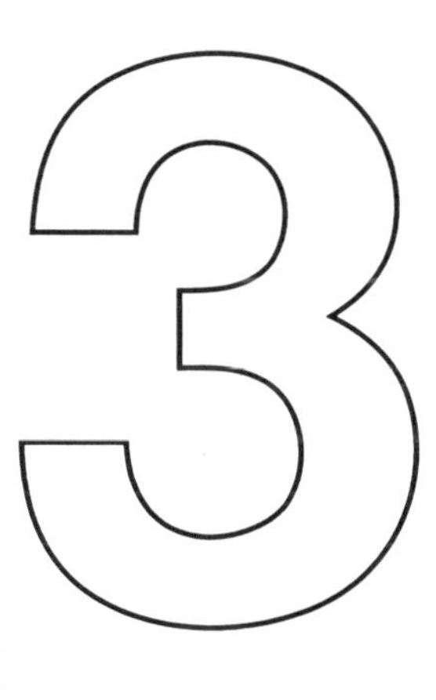

Model, Talk, Listen, Play

To young children, one of the most powerful attractions in the home is the television set. But that attraction doesn't just happen. If young children watch a lot of television, especially very young children, it's because they have learned that was what they were supposed to do. _Children learn this behavior from the parents._

Remember, when children are born they know nothing about television—or anything else. Their first experiences come from what they perceive at home. If the television is on all the time, they learn that is the usual state of affairs. If mother and father are watching, it must be okay—the thing to do. If no one stops the child from watching, then that too is okay. Young children will imitate what they see their parents do.

People often get upset about effects that television seems to have on children. We have all heard about the extent of television viewing, and feel somehow helpless to control this phenomenon.

It is true that the average child watches about seven thousand hours of television before entering kindergarten. Estimates indicate that young children log in approximately eleven thousand hours of television before they graduate from high school. But what does that all mean for your child? Is it good or bad? What should you do?

First of all, let's look at some of the data that have been reported in the past. This will be just a quick overview, and is not intended to be a complete synopsis. Many volumes have been written on each of these items, and you may want to read further later.

Numbers are always interesting, so let's begin there. We'll use averages and rounded numbers for purposes of illustration. Take the seven thousand hours in five years. That's only about four hours per day. I say *only* because many adults log that much time without giving it a second thought. A couple of sitcoms and a movie total four hours. Add a ball game, and you're way over that number. In fact, many surveys indicate that the average adult viewer watches beyond that amount. Five-plus hours of viewing per day is not uncommon. But, we'll stay with four hours per day.

What do young children see during that time? First we should look at the commercial messages. Most commercials are only fifteen seconds long with an average of six minutes of commercials per hour of programming. So, four hours of viewing, times six minutes of commercials per hour, times four commercials per minute totals 98 commercials per viewing day. Round that out to an even 100 and we can say the average four-hour-a-day viewer watches 700 commercials every week for a grand total of 36,500 commercials every year!

But what does this number have to do with *taking charge* of your child's education. On one hand, it's up to you to determine if you want your child to watch that many sales pitches. If not, turn off the television set. If you don't want to do that you will need to pay attention to what your child is learning. You should watch, too. If you can't do that, then you should plan to talk to your child about what he or she sees. Have your child describe what he or she watches. Ask her or him to decide if all the information is correct, or right, or fair, or some other description that he or she understands.

This leads us back to decision making.

There are two key factors here. Talk to the child, and model the behavior you want her or him to follow.

First, let's look at the behavior of talking. Ask your child what he or she sees and what he or she thinks about it. Children may have a great deal of difficulty distinguishing the difference between reality and fiction. Ask if your child thinks that the things he or she sees are real or made up. Point out errors when they develop.

You won't be able to do that, though, if you haven't watched the programs your child has. If you don't have information you won't be able to formulate appropriate questions. You'll be able to get a lot more out of the program than your child will, so lead your child to find answers that he or she will understand.

Modeling Behaviors

You can talk all you want about television viewing—or any other activity—but your child will do what you do. So determine what you want your child to do. Do you want your child to develop the habit of reading after dinner or before going to sleep? If you do it, your child will be much more likely to do the same.

After dinner, instead of turning on the television set, sit down and read a book, a magazine, or the newspaper. Just read, that's all. The specific material isn't as important as the *act of reading*. Your young child will see what you are doing and will want to do the same thing.

Your child may want to read what you are reading, and that will mean sitting next to you or on your lap. There is often a temptation to suggest that the child do something else to allow yourself time alone, but resist that temptation. Devote a few minutes to the child at this time, when the child's interest is aroused. Two things will happen. First, the child will enjoy the experience of being close to you and sharing this activity. Second, the time spent will probably pass very quickly.

A young child's attention span is rather short, and he or she will be off to some other activity pretty quickly. But, he or she should be the one to elect something else; the child should not feel forced to do something else because you didn't want to be bothered. The child knows that he or she has spent time in a very pleasant activity with you, and you liked it also. At least the child will be able to think so. Now, you can return to your own reading if you want.

When we discussed television viewing, we suggested that you talk to your child about what had been seen. Let's expand on that a bit.

Talking

Talk to your child as much as you can, and listen, too. Talking will expand the child's world greatly and help the child to do two things: acquire information, and then apply it. The new information is easily observed in an expanding vocabulary. There will be more words to use for more things in the child's environment. The names of things, places, people, and actions will become part of the child's spoken vocabulary, and the child will ask for and explain what he or she wants, feels, and needs.

It probably isn't necessary to say this in most instances, but we'll include it here anyway: *don't talk baby talk.* Talk like an adult. Use proper pronunciation and proper grammar.

Don't feel that inaccuracies or short cuts will make it easier for your child to understand what you are saying. Remember, the child is starting with a blank slate, and must learn everything from the beginning anyway. It's just as easy, or as difficult, to learn vocabulary, syntax, and grammar correctly as it is to learn it incorrectly. In fact, you do your child a favor when you emphasize and model the correct grammar and syntax right from the start. In that way the child will always have known and used the correct forms, and will never have to break bad habits, unlearn and then relearn. Proper modeling at this stage of the child's life will save a great deal of time and effort later.

Telling Stories

For practice of vocabulary, grammar, and syntax, tell stories. This can be the telling or retelling of a favorite story or fairy tale, or it can be telling about what happened to you when you were a child; places you visited, people you knew, games you played, or many other topics. The mere telling of the stories will give your child more practice in listening and, therefore, expanding vocabulary; and it will help in strengthening the important bond between parent and child. Through the storytelling, your child will learn more about you as a person in addition to knowing you as a parent.

Then turn the tables. Let your child tell you stories. These too can be favorite stories or tales about what the child did during the day. Children may even want to tell make-believe stories about great adventures they have had. Let them. It can be fun for them and for you. It can even provide an opportunity to focus on the differences between reality and fantasy, or fiction, so the children will grow to understand those differences. Of course, that increased understanding can also be applied when you talk about television programs, as well as about a specific story.

In later years when your child has acquired some of the necessary skills, you might want to write down these stories, or record them on audio or video tape. But for now, just enjoy the stories and the experience of sharing them as a family. This is part of *acquiring* the skills. The writing and recording will be part of *applying* them. We talked about those elements earlier.

When everyone takes part in this kind of activity it is truly sharing time. And your child's communication skills will get a good workout every day. That's great preparation for the school years yet to come.

This provides practice that isn't work. It's part of the daily routine in the family. Everyone does it so your child will simply be participating along with everyone else. What a wonderful way to practice: without evaluation, competition, or judgment.

Other Activities

Take your young children on visits and explorations. Do this in the neighborhood, at the store, at the park, or any place you have to go during the day. Take your child with you, and talk about the "wonders" that you see. This may sound a little silly to you, talking about the "wonders" of the supermarket, but remember, although it might not be a wonder to you, it probably will be to your child—if you let it be. Also, this activity isn't for your benefit anyway; it's for your child's benefit. So look for the wonder, and communicate it. This activity will also provide material for the storytelling times.

During the past few years, in ever increasing numbers, parents have been taking their young children to work with them. This activity was started in order to allow little girls to learn what their parents do during the day and to encourage the girls to aspire to jobs, occupations, and careers that once were not available to them.

When your child sees what you do, there will be a greater understanding of your day and there will be much more to talk about at home. More practice!

We have described some of these activities as though there were only two people involved: a parent and a child. Often there will be more than one of each participating. Two parents, perhaps a grandparent or other adult, and numerous siblings can participate at the same time. This greatly expands the opportunities and the topics available. It also provides insight into something you might find yourself thinking about in a few years when your child goes to school.

All the activities in which the family participates are carried out by a group that is *multi-age*. Well, you say, that's obvious. It is obvious, but most of us have never thought of it in exactly this way. We know that age differences exist between different adults, between different children, and certainly, between parents and their children. All the members of the family can take part in the same activity at the same time. Each member contributes differently, and each derives benefits to an extent different from the other group members. Although the group is multi-age and the experiences are different, the experiences are of benefit to each one, at her or his own level, and to the limit of her or his abilities. It's not necessary to set up different activities so that only people of the same age can participate at a particular time.

Multi-age groups are a part of our society. Families are multi-age; religious groups are multi-age; various social groups are multi-age. And all of those groups work.

What is the purpose of stressing what seems to be so obvious? Before long your child will enter an organization based heavily on age: he or she will enter school.

Over the years, the education system has been operated on the basis that age is extremely important. Children enter kindergarten at age 5, not 4, not 6, but only at age 5.

We all learn a great deal in multi-age groups so you may want to find out what your child's school thinks of multi-age grouping. We will discuss more about this subject in a later section.

In summary, what should you do at home? Several basic activities are significant:

- Model.
- Talk.
- Listen.
- Play an active role in your child's life.
- Be sure your child is a full participant in yours.

Toys   First of all—toys are for fun. Sometimes we adults get caught up with the notion that all toys must have some educational value. We feel that, somehow, kids should be learning something specific whenever they are occupied with a toy. Adults feel this way, but kids don't. That's why they will often open a package, remove the toy from inside, put the toy aside and play with the box. When that happens the child is exploring, imitating, and fabricating. The child is trying out observations and possibilities. Certainly the child is learning, but privately he or she is just having fun. The child is *playing*.

Selecting Toys   When you select toys, therefore, look for those that will encourage participation, and those that are fun. A suggestion, though: be sure the participation and fun will be positive and constructive. A gift of a cigarette lighter might be fun, but certainly it isn't constructive for a young child. Likewise, toy guns, knives, etc., should be avoided in favor of more constructive items such as blocks, cars, dolls, puzzles, and crayons.

What then should we look for? Human beings are attracted by many factors; primary among these elements are *light, color,* and *movement.* In selecting toys, keep those factors in mind. Will the color of the toy attract? Is it bright? Does it move?

Consider the toy in terms of safety. Will the colors come off? Will the pieces come apart?

Now consider what the toy does. Does it simply provide an attraction, something to look at? Does it invite the child to use it somehow? Build a building with blocks, drive a car, fly an airplane? Does it encourage the child to draw a picture, sculpt a statue, or play make-believe? Does it challenge the child to assemble a jigsaw puzzle or build a train?

In addition to the attraction of sight and movement, we should look for toys that appeal to other senses. What kinds of sounds do the toys make? What do they feel like?

Sounds can frighten, and they can comfort. Sudden, loud noises should be avoided when purchasing for a young child; soft, melodic items are usually beneficial— and are often treasured.

Likewise, hard, sharp objects are not nearly as pleasant to hold as those that are soft and round. In the vernacular, look for the "warm fuzzies."

Educational Toys

Toys can be "educational" in that they are *designed specifically to provide structured educational activities; but they certainly don't have to be.* All toys are educational in some way—they provide sensory experiences, practice for motor skills, or practice in arranging color or shape, etc. In selecting toys for young children, it is enough that the toy is safe, attractive, and interesting to the child. Give your child time, and pleasant toys, and the child will use the toys in a multitude of ways to develop many skills. As the child gets older, and has developed hand-eye coordination and other motor skills, more structured toys can be introduced, as the child is ready for them. But at no time should structured learning situations be expected to fill all the child's play time. The child's natural inclination to learn must be allowed some freedom through all growth stages, and the "luxury" of this free play time is often the most fertile and productive of the child's learning experiences.

There are so many toy items to choose from that it would be impossible to develop a definitive list of selections here. Furthermore, new toys appear so often that any such list would become obsolete very quickly. Perhaps the best guidelines can be provided through the application of the motto of the American Medical Association, *"Primum non Nocere"* which means "First of all, do no harm."

What Can We Expect from Toys?

Toys can be valuable in assisting children in the acquisition and development of a variety of concepts such as big–small, bigger–smaller, fast–slow, tall–short, ahead–behind, and many, many others.

Toys also help in the development of vocabulary because the child will want to know the names of parts of the toys and what the toys represent.

This development of concepts will play a significant role when the child goes to school and begins the early steps in learning to read. That might sound a bit strange, but here is what happens.

Early reading material, called "reading readiness" material, requires children to identify a number of different factors and to make selections from a number of options. For example, children are asked to, "mark the *biggest tree*" in a picture or, "Put an X in the *smallest box.*"

If children have not yet mastered the concepts of biggest and smallest, there is no way they can successfully carry out the required task. Schools include these concepts in their curriculum at the preschool and early childhood levels, but the child who understands them already has a decided advantage. Children who have not grasped them could be suspected of having a reading or learning disability which, in fact, might be traceable to just a gap in experiential learning.

Anxiety about this kind of performance can be prevented if children have plenty of opportunity for play experiences, and talk about their play, at home. Again "talk" practicing the communication skills at home is very important for your child. So help encourage your child with this every way you can.

This has been a long jump from toys to self-image, but there is a direct line, and we must be aware of it.

Since many toys are representational, it is possible for them to mimic the real world and, therefore, assist a child to expand her or his horizons within a controlled environment. Our ability to understand and transmit ideas is directly related to the extent of our working vocabulary, and toys add greatly to a child's list of words. Colors, shapes, textures, sounds, positions, quantities, movement, etc., all have names and as a child learns those names in playing with toys, it becomes a simple matter to transfer their use to the larger world.

The social and psychological benefits of toys are well known and used in therapy when necessary, so we won't try to explore that specialized area use. We will, however, suggest that observations of how a child plays with toys as well as the specific toys he or she prefers will provide insight into the child's abilities, likes, and fears.

Toys then are for fun, but also provide a firm foundation for the formation of concepts that will be used in intellectual or cognitive activities such as reading and mathematics. Further, they provide an outlet for the child as well as an observation platform for the adult who is interested in monitoring and guiding the child's growth and development.

It is also appropriate to mention again that learning the complex concepts we described earlier requires a great deal of effort. Toys, however, make such learning "fun" rather than "work." Because the association with toys is pleasurable, the time spent in play is extended, and children will focus attention and energy on their play without ever realizing how much they are learning.

As parents, we should seek out toys that help develop those concepts through play so that the child will be able to use them in future academic activities. We can relax, though, and enjoy buying toys that are "just for fun." These are often among the most productive in the child's learning environment—the most enduring and the most endearing.

Should I Buy a Computer?

What Do You Want to Do with a Computer?

A computer is a marvelous machine, one that will be in nearly every household in the not too distant future. There are other wonderful machines in our lives—television sets, radios, automobiles, and hundreds of other devices. In selecting any of these the first question we must ask relates to intent. What do we want them to do for us? Why do we need them?

In thinking about the purchase of a computer, if the primary reason you are interested in buying it is to assure that your young child gets into college, please think again.

There have been many commercials on television designed to play on the fears of parents by telling and showing them how disappointed their children will be when they have to return home from college because they were unprepared for the academic tasks that awaited them. If only they had had a computer, things would have been different! Viewers are told not to let this happen to their children. "Buy Brand X Computer, and your child's future will be assured!" they would like us to believe. Nonsense!

Computers, like all other machines, are tools and that's all they are. How much we get out of them depends on how we use them.

This is not to say that the computer is not a very important tool in our society; without a doubt, it is, and it is becoming more so with each year. We will want our children to know how to use them, and when our children are young, we ourselves will want to know how to guide our children in using them well.

Computers can be very expensive, so remember it is not necessary to buy a computer for use in your own home. Many alternatives exist: public and parochial schools include computer use at early grades, in most areas. Even if your schools do not have computers available for young children's use, most major public libraries have computers available. The computers designed for young children's use are usually located in the children's literature department, or in a separate computer area. Librarians can direct you to persons on the staff who will instruct you and your children in using the computers and the various kinds of software that the library has available. Familiarity with the use of computers is thus available without the expense of purchasing a computer for your home.

Should You Introduce Your Young Child to Computer Use, and If So, When?

Readiness is all, they say, and this applies to computer use as well as to use of any other tool. Very young children, up to about ages three and four years, may not yet have developed enough small muscle control to enjoy using a computer or any other machine that has small parts to be manipulated for any length of time. It stands to reason that if your child likes to sit for extended periods of time, playing with crayons, paints, pens and pencils, or your old typewriter, you can assume that the child will be ready to play with appropriate software programs on the computer. Software programs exist for children as young as three and four years of age, and most of these have been developed carefully for the capabilities of these children.

Most current software programs, for example, incorporate pictures in the menu, and young children do not need to know how to read in order to use such programs. Games are made up to help the young child become familiar with the keyboard, and to have fun with letters and numbers, matching games, counting, adding and subtracting in pictures, manipulating pictures of blocks on the screen and similar simple games. A wide variety of computer games is usually available at your public library, so you and your young child can practice using the computer, and see how you do. If the activity is not an enjoyable one for both you and your child, once you have become familiar with the use of the machine, wait a few months, and see if your child enjoys the activity more then.

Deciding When and If You Want to Buy a Computer

Before you plan to buy a computer for your young children to use at home, it is a good idea to try out such programs, and see for yourself whether or not your child is ready for them. Computer manufacturers put out booklets that describe their programs, and most list the age levels for which the programs are appropriate. Remember though, these age levels are general guidelines. These guidelines may or may not match with your child.

If they don't, there isn't anything wrong with your child or with the guidelines. They just don't match—that's all.

If you have tried out a few software programs, and found that your child enjoys the activity, then you may want to consider buying a computer for the child's use at home. At that point, you should examine several different kinds of computers to see which one you and your child like to use most. Computer stores are usually more than willing to demonstrate the computer's capabilities and allow you time to play with the machines under their guidance.

Your selection should be made on the basis of which computers have available the kinds of software that you want to use. Software programs for children from ages three to five are primarily nonverbal, and use many visuals in the games they supply. From age six up, the programs are more complex, using more reading skills, and more mathematics skills, in line with the skills the children are learning in school.

Programs are available that are highly imaginative, and provide opportunities for children to explore the capabilities of the computer program, as well as to explore their own use of verbal and mathematical skills, and other skills such as sequencing, logical arrangement, manipulation of shapes, patterns, movement, etc. There are also programs that provide rote drill to practice such skills as spelling, reading, writing, mathematic, science, social studies, and the like. The former are usually more fun to use, including as they do more novelty, surprise, imaginative visuals, and elements such as competition, or puzzles. The latter, the "skill drill" type, may also be very imaginative, and it is fair to say you should judge each program individually; but they *may* be more monotonous, and provide for far less in the way of creative use by the young child. In keeping with our earlier thoughts, they might not be very much "fun" either. If that's the case you have to wonder if your child will ever use it.

Another point to remember if you think that you may want to select some "skill drill" software for your child is that it is a good idea to talk over the project with your child's teacher or teachers, and invite them to tell you their thoughts on software use. If programs are already in use in the school, the teacher's input can save you time and money in letting you know what the child already has available. Also, if the teacher can fill you in on the skill areas that would be beneficial for your child to practice, you can be that much more specific in choosing software programs.

You should set up a file or a notebook to jot down your growing amount of information about software programs, and list the names that you try out so that you can remember which ones you liked and which ones you didn't. Once you have established what kinds of software you would like to use, at least to begin with, then you will be ready to start making the decision of what machine to buy.

Deciding What Machine to Buy

Your choice of a personal computer will be based on: What software do you foresee using, and with which machines is this software compatible? Of this group of machines, which one offers the best buy for the money?

At this point you will want to visit more than one computer store, and perhaps more than one software supplier. Try out machines within your price range, and even some that are a bit over. See what software is available for the machines you like best. Ask for the manufacturers' booklets on their software, and their machines, and study these before you make a decision. Collect all the information you can from friends, teachers, business acquaintances, and computer sales people. Ask which machines have the most appropriate software for your purposes, and which are compatible with other manufacturers' software, and also with other manufacturers' components. If you want to have a printing capability for your own use or your child's, be sure you compare the quality of various printer components, and decide what quality you really want.

If you are planning to use the computer for recreation, family business, household record keeping, as well as for young child's play and learning activities, you will want to make this clear to the dealer, and be sure that the machine has a good memory capability, as well as a good printer, and good compatibility with a variety of software.

Most manufacturers supply booklets that are exact and specific, and although it is time-consuming to read them thoroughly, it will be well worth the time and effort when you invest in your computer.

A Final Word

Remember that learning—real learning—is fun. If your young child shows resistance to the use of the computer, it is best to wait, and try again at six-month intervals until the child seems more receptive. If the use of the computer is fun for the child from the beginning, your next task may be to see that he or she doesn't take over the machine and become as fixated on it as some children have done with television! Try to maintain a balance of time used with the computer, just as you do with the television, or any other device. Balance the kinds of software that you make available, too. No one wants to spend hours at "drill and skill" exercises, and since your objective is to further your child's enjoyment of the learning process, you will be able to tell if the drills are defeating their purpose.

For additional information on kinds of software programs and what they have to offer, refer to magazines that offer reviews and evaluations of software and hardware. Because of the fast growth in this field, you will find that your public library or local bookstore has many such periodicals to offer. In addition, the American Library Association publishes *Book List,* which is a highly respected periodical for professional librarians and others who select and buy materials. This publication offers reviews of new computer software, and evaluates the products. *School Library Journal* also publishes reviews of books and software for young people. Ask the librarian at your library or school for these materials.

Appendix B at the end of this book provides additional guidelines and resources for you to use in judging types of computer programs and computer hardware. It will help you to distinguish between drill and skill materials, interactive materials, and the hardware you will need to use these programs. As software and hardware are developed in increasing variety, you will have much from which to choose.

Finally, if you feel that buying a computer would be good for you and your young child, that is the best reason to buy it, not because of a neighbor's urging, or the urging of commercials you see on television. If you're not sure, wait awhile and do more investigating; your child won't flunk out of school if you don't buy a computer right away—regardless of what the commercials may say!

Getting Your Child Ready to Learn at School

"The parent and the school are partners: The parent sets the pattern, and the school must take what it gets."

This old saying illustrates the position of our schools in some ways, when they receive students and prepare to teach them.

As we have said earlier, each child enters the family world like a blank slate. There is relatively little written there yet, but anything and everything can be recorded on that surface in the course of just a few short years. The school, on the other hand, is presented with a child whose personality, attributes, and learning habits are partially developed. The child is no longer a blank slate, but comes equipped with likes, dislikes, expectations, and an accumulation of experiences. And the school must work with the child in whatever forms and states of readiness for learning that exist.

One of the greatest gifts a parent can give a child is the desire to learn. Skills and specific content will come later in many forms, but they will be evident only to the extent that the child wants to acquire new information. What a child thinks and feels about school and learning in general usually is directly related to the conditioning the child has received at home.

Parents have several years in which to establish and nurture a desire to learn. The results of the early years at home with the parents are reflected in how a growing child feels about schooling later. The child's attitude will be either positive or negative. The learning process will be viewed as fun, exciting, worthwhile, stimulating, and positive; or it will be seen as boring, frightening, useless, and negative.

The Role of Parents

An interesting study was conducted in the mid-1960s. Researchers wanted to find out if and how parents conditioned their children toward the learning process and, therefore, toward going to school. They wanted to see if parents did anything special that would encourage or discourage children from learning, so they set up the following experiment.

Parents and their young preschool children were the participants. For the most part, the parent was the mother rather than the father; but there was an even distribution of boys and girls.

The experiment consisted of having the parent teach a specific task to her or his child using any verbal directions he or she wanted. The only limitation in the study was that the parent could not demonstrate the task. She had to *tell* the child what to do.

The task consisted of arranging a set of blocks in a specified pattern on each of four equal sections on a board. A two-foot square board had been divided into four quadrants; blocks of different sizes, shapes, and colors had to be arranged in a predetermined pattern. The parent was taught the task by a researcher, and then the parent had to teach the child how to arrange the block. That's really all there was to it.

One by one each parent took her or his child into the testing room to teach the task. Researchers watched through a one-way mirror and recorded the language used by the parent.

After all the parents and children had been observed, the results of the teaching fell into two categories. One style reflected a very positive attitude toward learning and the other a very negative one. Here's what happened.

Within the negative group, almost all the directions from the parents were negative. "You aren't paying attention." "You aren't listening." "Don't look over there." "Don't talk back to me." "This isn't a time to play." Don't, Don't, Don't, No, No.

The other group, however, was very positive in approaching the task. The mother usually "set the scene" by referring to other similar situations like, "Remember when we played that game of blocks at your cousin's house? Well, this is a lot like that." Then the comments were very positive and reinforcing. "Very good." "You got that one right." "You are doing very well."

The conclusions derived from the experiment were quite dramatic. The children in the negative group did very poorly. They took a long time to complete the task in comparison to the other group. In fact, many children in the negative group didn't even finish. They cried and knocked the pieces off the board. The task was frustrating and unpleasant.

The other group, however, did quite well. Those children finished, and finished quickly. They saw the task as a game, as fun. The parent was a helper and a guide rather than a critic.

Because of the negative or positive attitudes of the parents, learning a simple task was frustrating or it was fun. And, observably, it was the parent who made the difference.

If, during the early years, children repeatedly experience negative feelings and directions when attempting to learn a task, their attitude toward learning in general becomes negative. Learning is seen as unpleasant, even painful; so why should children put themselves in such a negative situation? If, however, learning is perceived as fun, interesting, and pleasurable, a child will seek out such activities, and participate gladly. Learning itself is fun, and accomplishment provides extra rewards.

When "negative-oriented" children enter school they already know they don't want to be there. They know the experience will probably be painful, and that they won't do very well. They would clearly rather be someplace else doing something else.

"Positive-oriented" children, however, are eager, interested, and active. They want all they can get!

Imagine the task of the teacher when confronted by those two types of children: one child will most likely become an achiever. The other just might become a discipline problem. It certainly isn't difficult to guess which one is which. It isn't difficult to predict which child will benefit from the school years.

The role in which the child is cast is not her or his doing. The child didn't decide to be "positive" or "negative," didn't set out to establish a particular reputation.

According to the cited study, it was the way in which the parent *talked* to the child that determined what the attitude toward the learning task would be in later years. The manner in which the parent talked during the experiment was the way the parent usually talked to the child. No specific directions were given to the parent about what to say or not to say, so the parent simply talked in the "usual" manner.

During the formative years, each child comes to see learning as positive or negative depending on how her or his parents set up the conditions. A clear message is written on that blank slate, and the child then carries that message to school—maybe to other learning situations for the rest of her or his life.

The implications are clear. The way parents talk to young children about things related to learning has a profound effect on how children view learning in general and on how they approach formal education when they reach school age.

Parents, be careful about how you give directions and how you guide your child. Be positive in the language you use and in the directions and feedback you provide. This is another illustration of the old adage, "As the twig is bent, so grows the tree."

If, from their earliest recollections, your child sees learning as pleasurable, he or she will look forward to going to school and will probably do well there. The establishment of this positive attitude is basically up to you. It is your choice and your responsibility to create and maintain it.

You will also want to be sure that the learning environments in day care centers, preschools, and kindergarten are positive and encouraging to your young child. If negative teaching methods are used, it is important to identify and correct them quickly. If you are unsure, make arrangements to observe classes or play periods. Ask questions, without being accusing or irritable. If you find that your child is not receiving positive reinforcement, discuss the problem with the individual teacher, in private. Explain your feelings, and ask specifically for the change that you want. If the teacher can make the change, and does, you will have made good, quick improvement in the situation. If it seems that the teacher cannot make the change, then discuss the question with the school administration. Don't let weeks of precious time go by, hoping that things will improve by themselves. In a young child's life, weeks are a long time. Be prepared to make a change in schools if it is absolutely necessary, so that you do not feel desperate in the interview. Remember, even the school teachers and administrators will learn best in a positive environment, and you can make your point best by maintaining an attitude of positive expectation in your conversations with them.

The partnership between parent and teacher will produce positive results if the parent sets up the conditions for the teacher to develop. Neither partner can accomplish the task in isolation, but together they can have a significant effect on the life of a young child.

Specific Skills that Will Help Your Child in School

There are certainly many skills that will be helpful to your young child in beginning school, and a few guidelines on what to expect at certain ages.

If you are enrolling your child in a nursery school, it may be necessary to have the child toilet trained before the nursery school will admit her or him. Schools in this group usually have a minimum age requirement of two- to two-and-a-half years, as well. If your child is not yet used to using the toilet, it is not a good idea to force the issue just to make a deadline of getting the child into the nursery school. A better solution is to locate a day care center that accepts younger children, and is prepared to deal with them. Here, too, you will want to make sure that the day care center is positive in its teaching methods, and provides unstressful instructions for the children to follow.

If your child is toilet-trained, and is also comfortable with being away from you for several hours at a time, it is time to consider nursery school or preschool. Help your child get ready for this experience with visits to the school, during which the child can play with other children, make the acquaintance of teachers, and in effect *practice* for brief visits. This will give you a chance to observe your child's interest and degree of comfort in the school as well as to observe how the teacher and the aides behave toward and treat the children as a group and as individuals. At home, you can teach the child to hang up coats, put away boots and mittens, and get dressed to go outside.

Cognitive skills, such as learning vocabulary, the child's own name, and how to greet others, will also be of help at this age.

At about three-and-a-half to four years of age, you can usually expect young children to be interested in learning the concepts and the vocabulary of color, shape, size, odor, taste, texture, sounds, and positions. You can use these words and concepts in everyday situations at home or on excursions to the park, the zoo, and the like. Simply talking to, and with, your young children will help them develop these observational and vocabulary skills. Some simple examples of natural situations in which these conversations can occur are:

1. To help the child learn colors, ask if the child prefers a red crayon or a blue one; if he or she would like to put all the yellow napkins on the table, or get new green shoelaces when you make a shopping trip.

2. To learn shapes, let the child trace around objects to make pictures, and talk about the shapes as the child traces. Round jar lids, square pieces of cardboard, triangular blocks, oval soap bars, and rectangular shoe boxes all provide useful shapes to talk about.

3. Texture is fun to talk about, and easy to find in your own home: soft puppy fur, rough sandpaper, hard stones and bricks, slippery wet soap and the like are handy, and will amuse your young child.

4. Odors are funny sometimes, and you can play a game of letting the child identify favorite foods by their odors. Grape, cherry, and orange flavors are strong, and easily identified. Let your child close her or his eyes, and guess what juice is in the glass

for lunch today. Ketchup, mustard, oatmeal, pancake syrup, hotdogs, broccoli, and onions, all have distinctive odors, and guessing games will make it fun to identify them.

5. Tastes come in sweet, sour, bitter, and salty. Sometimes these are difficult even for adults to distinguish, because they are so often in combination. Pick the ones that are relatively simple, so the young child experiences success in naming them. Salt on pretzels, syrup or fruit, lemon juice or dill pickles, are easy to name as salt, sweet, and sour respectively. Bitter is harder, but there may be an occasion to take medicine, or lick an envelope that has a bitter tasting glue, and you can talk about all of these.

6. Sound is wonderfully complicated. You can start with loud and soft. Then try names of kinds of sounds: whistles, singing, barking, meowing, talking, calling, shouting, strumming, drumming, and on and on through whatever sounds are all around you for your child to enjoy. You can make use of the nursery rhymes and songs that mimic the sounds of drums, violins, and flutes, or birds, or goldfish in the water. Many children's books use sound in poetry and rhymes, and you can enjoy the sharing of the patterns of sounds as you read aloud to your child.

7. Positions include high, low, beside, close to, around, over, under, near, far, in back of, in front of, and at about age five or six, right and left. Simply using these words, and listening when your child uses them, is the best and most enjoyable way to teach your child their uses.

Some additional vocabulary skills will be helpful, including how to tell if things are alike or different; the same or not the same. On a visit to the zoo, you can ask your child to point out to you two animals that look the same, or two that are different from each other, in color, shape, size, or texture. At home, you can put two objects in a pillow case, and let your child feel them to see if they are the same or different. Let your child play the game with you, too, and hide two objects in the pillow case for you to guess. Matching socks, mittens, or colors of accessories when dressing can also provide this kind of useful game.

Counting games can start with one, two, three. When your child gets the idea, you will be asked, "How many is this?" "How many are there?" With children of three, four, and even five, you can introduce the names of numerals up to ten. Then let your child guide you in the introduction of higher numbers, when he or she is ready to ask about and learn them.

Let's Look at Preschools

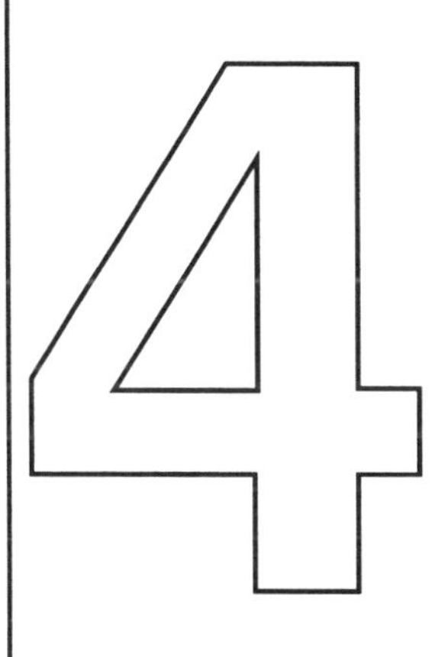

What Are Preschools?

As the name indicates, these are places parents send their children before the children are old enough to go to regular school. Regular school usually isn't available to children until they are at least 5 years old.

Preschools exist because parents can't—or choose not to—keep their young children at home all day before the law requires them to be in school. A variety of pressures in our society often makes it necessary and appropriate for both parents to be out of the house during the day. Our mobile society has likewise resulted in families that are separated geographically much of the day. Grandparents, aunts, and uncles, are no longer available to care for the child when the parents must be away, so another option had to be found. Preschools entered the picture.

Another important impetus to the preschool movement was the heightened awareness of the public in the 1960s of the potential for children's increased learning, especially in cognitive areas, if they received instruction and practice in basic skills earlier than age five or six. The preschool movement of the 1960s brought the term *learning objective* into the public eye, and parent groups, television, popular magazines, and other media began to inform the public about what educational and other experts thought about early childhood education.

The Headstart Program was an important educational effort at that time, and grew rapidly under the sponsorship of the federal government. Though funding later decreased, and the program diminished, tests showed that educationally the Headstart Program made significant differences in later school scores for many children. The influence of the curriculum that was developed during these years continues to be felt. The names of experts in the fields of education, and educational and child psychology, such as Carl Rogers and Jean Piaget, became familiar to parents and teachers, and an increased understanding of what young children could learn, and how they learned it at different stages, grew rapidly.

A sequence of basic skills involving the concepts of observation, comparison, description, grouping, and change was developed, and the best of the preschools have incorporated these curriculum areas into their programs at the preschool levels. Appropriate games and activities for individual children, small groups, and large groups were developed to help children develop these skills. An increased awareness in the public at large motivated commercial toy and educational materials companies to supply products that provided learning opportunities. The famous television program, *Sesame Street,* incorporated these skill areas, and was a pioneer in their use for television programming. Many others followed, both on public and network television channels.

Preschools in the public and private sectors gradually had available to them a rich variety of media to use in teaching young children—games, puzzles, television, video tape, and computer programs.

Not only the cognitive areas of learning were affected. The *affective* learning domain (that's education jargon—it relates to feelings and emotions) was incorporated as well, and the learning activities include those that provide young children with opportunity to observe and describe behavior in such areas as honesty, fairness, and cooperation.

With the demonstrated success of such curriculum content for children at the three-, four-, and five-year-old age levels, the preschool movement was strengthened greatly, and parents and the public at large have given increased support to the idea of early learning programs.

Sesame Street

Sesame Street continues to be a model of what "educational television" *can* be. It is still the standard by which other children's programs are measured.

Presently, there is another strong move by both private and public agencies to "require" all television stations to produce and air programs for young children. Those requirements go so far as to direct how many hours per day or week the stations must offer such programs.

On the surface that looks like a pretty good idea. The problem, however, is the definition of "educational" as well as the "requirement" to program for a specific audience for a specified amount of time.

In the past, stations have sometimes identified sitcom programs as "educational" just because they contained some subject matter that could be described as containing a "lesson" about life and/or getting along with peers. That has been a big stretch, but in some cases the stations got away with that reasoning.

If, indeed, we do see these new requirements take hold, be cautious. There is no substitute for *your* judgment. You can't afford to let a government agency or a station program director decide what is "good" for your young child.

The responsibility is yours. A law or a rule from the Federal Communications Commission doesn't necessarily mean the outcome is a good one. You must be on watch at all times.

You decide what is good for your child.

You decide what you want to make available in your home.

We'll deal more with television in another section of this book, but for now remember your young child will follow *your* direction. If you turn on and watch the television every day so will your child; if you watch "junk" so will your child. You will know it's junk, but will your child?

Are All Preschools the Same?

Absolutely not! Some provide instruction in a wide variety of areas, and some provide little more than custodial care. Some are strictly babysitting facilities.

If you become interested in sending your young child to a day care facility use great care in making the choice.

What Happens in Preschool?

Let's look first at the facilities that provide an instructional curriculum. They range from the well known, international Montessori Schools to locally controlled and independently operated programs in many locales.

In these institutions, children receive instruction in many of the basic skills: reading, writing, and mathematics. In many respects, these preschools provide much of the instruction that was once relegated to the primary, first, second, and third grades of elementary school.

As we began to realize that formal education didn't have to start only after age 5 or 6, there was an increased interest on the part of parents in having their children start learning earlier. The children were capable so the parents provided the opportunity.

A caution: if your child has had a stimulating experience in a preschool that provided academic instruction, pay attention to the curriculum of the kindergarten he or she attends at age 5. If the kindergarten does little more than repeat what has already been done in preschool, the child could quickly get bored and turn off to school. You cannot assume that the formal school system will automatically offer more challenges and opportunities than those that were available in preschool.

You will want to observe and ask questions early in your child's school career. In fact, start asking before your child is even old enough to enter school. Take some time to visit the kindergarten your child will attend. Call the school, and schedule visitation times. Talk to the teacher or teachers and to other parents about what the children do in kindergarten.

You will want to be sure that your child's education, which began long before the child entered school, continues in a good development sequence. Neither you nor your child has the time to repeat what is unnecessary.

Custodial Care

In custodial care centers, children are simply cared for. Their social and physical needs are provided for. Custodial care facilities concentrate on the physical well being of the child. Their primary reason for existence is to assure the comfort and safety of children when parents must be away from them.

Little emphasis is given to teaching, although there is usually some instruction in art, music, and painting. Children will do things and make things, but it is the physical rather than the intellectual care and development that is stressed.

As with instructional facilities, the sophistication of these custodial care facilities varies greatly. There are some that belong to nationwide chains, and others that are one-of-a-kind independent operations. The quality of each kind can vary.

The national organizations usually have a well developed curriculum, and are well monitored by a professional staff. Their operations are extensive and they are careful about maintaining the quality of their facilities. Ask about the affiliation of the preschool you are visiting. If it is part of a larger company, ask to see literature including annual reports as well as promotional material.

The quality of small, independent operations varies widely. Some are excellent, but others leave a great deal to be desired. They are usually individually owned, and most are owned and operated by women. They are often located in populated areas where there is a great need for day care for the children of working parents, and there may be less emphasis on learning.

Some of these are operated in houses and, in many instances, store fronts. Variation in quality of care is so broad that only careful examination can determine how well a particular facility will care for your child. You will want to be sure to visit all the places you are considering. Again, ask about affiliation, the training of the staff, what the children actually do in the facility, the names of parents you can contact for more information, and ask to see evaluative reports that may have been submitted by outside agencies. Also, go visit the facility more than once.

Call to set up the first visit, but don't hesitate to "drop in" sometime. You just might find a substantial difference in what you see in an expected visit and an unexpected one. Now, this in itself shouldn't surprise you too much, because we all take care to prepare for visitors, even at home, but look for vast differences. It is absolutely essential to be cautious about places where you leave your child, even when it is a school. You certainly wouldn't turn your child over to a stranger on the street or in the supermarket. The staff of a preschool is made up of strangers until you know a substantial amount about them.

Start looking around early. Don't wait until you have an urgent need for a place to send your child. A hasty decision in this area just shouldn't be made.

Infant Care

Some facilities specialize in the care of very young children, infants, and toddlers; their facilities are usually designed specifically for children who still need a great deal of personal care and assistance.

These places are usually small and provide for only a dozen or so children at a time. They usually provide care and feeding functions, and that's all. They are places parents can leave their babies and assume that they will be cared for. But, please don't assume too much. Visit. Ask questions. Be sure the staff is responsible, gentle, and responsive to the children as individuals.

Set up the visits the same way we suggested in the section on custodial care facilities, and ask the same questions.

Licensing

There are some licensing requirements for preschools, but much of the criteria for licensing is based on the physical facilities rather than on the programs or the personnel. Licensing factors focus on such things as square footage of work space, playground, rest areas, toilet facilities, etc.

In most areas, the people who work in preschool facilities are not required to have specific training or preparation. Only the director of the center must be able to show that a few specific courses were taken, often no more than a community college program; no degree is required, and no certification examination or review must be completed or passed.

Because of our backgrounds and experiences, we often assume that anyone working in any kind of a school is certified to do so. This is just not the case. The type of certification and training required of public school teachers simply does not exist for preschool operators.

How to Pick a Preschool

Your first contact should be the State Board of Education. Some state boards of education maintain liaisons with other education-related agencies, and they can often give specific advice on certain facilities. Preschools that try to offer quality programs usually seek out the cooperation of such state agencies and try to provide stimulating opportunities for children. But, the state covers a great deal of territory so you will also want to look to local agencies for help.

The first such agency is the local school district. Local school districts are not in competition with most preschools. On the contrary, the local schools are the recipients of the output of the preschools so they are in an excellent position to comment on what the preschools do.

Teachers at all levels of education who receive students from other schools often comment that it is possible to tell what previous schools in the area students attended before entering the new schools. Elementary school teachers often are aware of the differences that can be expected from various preschools. Schedule a meeting with the principal and kindergarten teachers in your local school. Your child may eventually attend that school so you will have an opportunity to start to learn about it and the staff, as well as to investigate the local preschool reputations.

Ask questions about the preschools in the neighborhood including the following:

Can you tell what preschool your new students attended?

What characteristics enable you to tell?

Will you list the preschools from best to worst?

What elements do you consider most important in determining best and worst?

What can I expect my child to do in each school?

What should I expect my child to get out of preschool in the first place?

Should I send my child to preschool at all?

What kind of disadvantage will my child bring to school if he or she doesn't go to a preschool first?

If I have to be away all day, is there a recommended variety of activities, programs, or schools I should consider, or will one place provide all my child will need?

What kinds of problems has the community had with any of the different preschools?

Have you had meetings with the preschool teachers?

If you haven't met—why not? Is there any special reason for the lack of contact between preschools and primary grade schools?

Can you recommend other sources of information?

If you live in an area where there is a higher education institution, check to see if it offers an early childhood program. Many colleges, universities, and community colleges with teacher training institutions offer such programs, and the college personnel are well informed about the preschools in their areas. The faculties usually visit the preschools regularly, and the graduates seek employment in existing preschools or they establish their own. These college faculty members will likely be able to discuss various programs in general, but they may hesitate to give specific recommendations or criticisms unless there is exceptional reason to do so. But listen for the tone of their comments.

You will want to consider the following points in your interviews with these professionals:

- Is there any hesitation about commenting on the value of a specific preschool?

- Is there a lack of information about a specific preschool that might indicate a closed operation?

- Does the faculty member volunteer information and comments about specific preschools? If so, probe. Ask the follow-up questions: Why do you say that? How can you be sure of that?

Ask the college faculty member for a list of preschools in the area that you might visit. Through such a simple request you might discover options you were previously unaware of, or you might find that preschools you were considering are not included on the list. If that's the case, ask specifically about those. It simply might have been overlooked, or it might have been omitted deliberately. In either case, your probe will help you decide where to place your child.

Next, check other local agencies like the Health Department, Children and Family Services, and maybe even the Better Business Bureau. Those agencies will be in a position to advise you on the service and business reputations of the various preschools in the area that you are considering.

Often we focus on the intellectual, social, and physical elements of the preschool and overlook the fact that the preschool is a business, a business that provides a service. We should, therefore, be just as interested in how well a preschool conducts its business as we are in the quality of its service. You will want to find out about the following factors:

- How well does it meet regulatory requirements including fire safety codes, health code expectations, etc.? Is it licensed?
- Does it pay its bills on time?
- What kind of financial support does it receive?
- In addition to tuition, where does its money come from? Grants? State or federal funding? Religious groups? Others?
- Is it "not-for-profit" or "for profit"?
- Who controls the programs, personnel, etc.?
- Are the employees from the community or from elsewhere? Does this affect the quality of the program in any way? How?

Since preschools are businesses, remember that two major questions should be asked concerning any business operation: Who does the work? And, where does the money come from?

This list of suggested questions for a variety of organizations and agencies might seem to be overly extensive. But, that is exactly why you should carry out such an investigation. You are going to turn your child over to a stranger in a strange location. Your goal is to eliminate— or certainly minimize—the unknown quantities and qualities. The time your child will spend in the preschool is a nonrenewable commodity. What happens there will affect the rest of her or his life. Although that might sound a bit dramatic, it's absolutely true. Every experience we have affects our entire lives, and a great many experiences will be included during the days, weeks, months, and years your child is in the care of teachers and other staff members in preschool.

The Corporate Preschool

One final comment about preschools. Many employers now offer preschools on site in order to make it more convenient for parents to provide care for their young children, as well as to continue to work. In such cases, the employer has usually investigated the teachers carefully and is sure the program offerings will be positive. You will still wish to visit the site and ask some of these same questions, however, to determine if the program provides what you want for your child. We have discussed some of the differences that exist in programs so be sure that your place of business matches what you want. Convenience can be a very important consideration, but you don't want to let it automatically outweigh the other important factors we have considered.

Choices: Public or Private

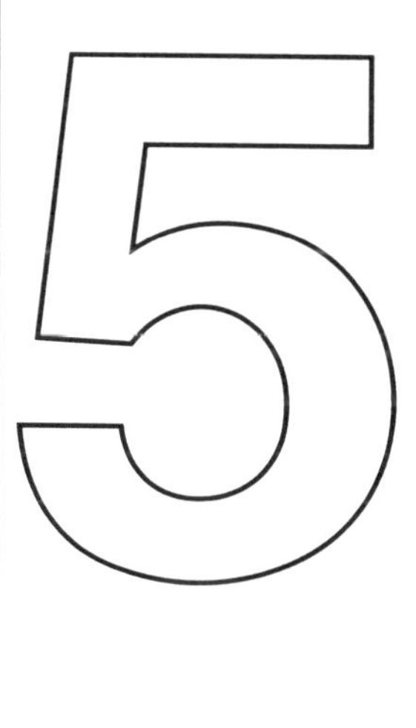

Choosing for Kindergarten or First Grade

Before your child reaches age five or six, you will want to plan what school he or she will attend, beginning with kindergarten or first grade.

Deciding what type of school—public or private—will be best for your child can be the easiest or the most difficult decision you face at this early stage of your child's education.

What factors will make it easy? First, money. Public schools are free, private schools require tuition.

The ease of that decision, however, might change if some current discussions ever come to fruition. Paying tuition currently can cause such a severe hardship on many families that private education is out of the question. There is periodic debate in various legislatures proposing an answer to that problem by making exceptions to the current funding rules.

schools. That would result in a widening class distinction between the private school students and the public school students. One of the major purposes of American schools—the education of a diverse population—would disappear.

Watch the papers for further developments.

Family Tradition

Another reason that private schools could be an easy choice is family tradition. Some families have traditionally sent their children to private schools, and you might plan to continue that tradition. This is often true, of course, in the case of parochial schools. When ethnic or religious preferences are taken into consideration, parents frequently send their children to the schools where appropriate social, language, or religious training will be an integral part of the program. When that is the case, most other considerations are minimized in favor of the overriding one of cultural or religious affiliation.

Let's assume for the moment, however, that you are undecided about private versus public schools.

There are many people who feel that private is better, period. This assumption is not necessarily so.

What factors should you consider—other than cost?

Private School Programs

Is the overall course of study appropriate for a broad spectrum of the population or is it designed for a very narrow segment? Where does your child fit in that range?

The public school, by definition, is designed to appeal to the general public. It is intended to provide a broad general opportunity to everyone. Obviously, there is little chance for providing special consideration to individuals within that broad population—with two notable exceptions.

Gifted Programs

Gifted children, those with exceptional abilities in certain areas, may receive consideration above and beyond what is offered to the average child. Many schools offer gifted programs in which academic, artistic, and athletic abilities are often enhanced. These gifted programs are usually offered within the elementary school, but sometimes are provided in specially designated facilities. Children who take part in the gifted program may be bused to another building at some distance.

Admission to these programs is often determined through teacher recommendation, testing, audition, or some other form of performance. The specifics of the admission process are determined by the area of concentration, population, and degree of competition.

Funding is provided by the board of education although parents are often expected to provide some assistance in the form of financial support, for example, paying for transportation. Some federal and state funding is available for gifted programs, so although the local board of education is the responsible party, there is outside assistance available.

Special Education

Special education is the other area of the public school offering that focuses on a specified, select population. Special education usually refers to programs for students with some type of handicap or disability. These include physical, mental, emotional, and social disabilities.

By law, public schools must provide appropriate educational opportunities for all children. For those students who are unable to function in the regular classroom, arrangements are made to provide for them elsewhere. These requirements may be met in separate classrooms within a public school building, or appropriate care and education may be possible only in specifically designed and operated facilities.

Most school systems today implement "inclusion." Inclusion simply means that all children are included in the regular classrooms to the fullest extent possible.

Children needing special, separate attention and facilities will receive them, but wherever possible they will be placed in regular classrooms.

There is some controversy over inclusion that you should think about. Some people feel that it slows down the pace in what otherwise would be a "normal" classroom. If some of the children cannot work at a "normal" pace, the other children will suffer.

On the other hand, for the "special child" the daily association with the "normal" children will serve as an incentive.

This book is not the place to take a position on the issue or to attempt to describe inclusion in detail. I bring it up here so you will think about it and its impact on your young child. It makes no difference if your child is in the "normal" category or the "special" category—inclusion *will* have an effect on your child's education.

Severely mentally handicapped children, for example, require attention beyond what can be provided by a regular classroom teacher. The same might be true for children with severe physical disabilities. Rather than deprive such children of educational opportunities because they cannot function within the confines of the regular classroom, special arrangements are made and provided by the public schools.

If your child requires such attention you will probably be concerned with cost, but you don't have to be. These special programs are funded by the local school district with assistance from the state and federal governments. Such special care will not add to the cost of educating your child even if the services are provided in a special classroom, or at a distant facility. Expenses are paid by the local district. Ask your school board or school administration about this if you have need for such services.

It is clear, then, that certain groups of students with special needs are given special consideration in public schools; such consideration is not usually available through private schools except at a very high cost. Parents of children with these special needs should look first to the public schools for appropriate programs that won't create a financial burden.

Special Public Schools

In an effort to intensify the offerings of the public schools, many district are reorganizing their schools. They are creating schools that concentrate on specific areas of interest that might include academics, music, the performing arts, etc. Such schools are known by a variety of names including Magnet Schools and Laboratory Schools. They are funded and operated by the local district. If there is one in your district, you might wish to consider what it can offer your child—as well as what will be expected of you.

Although children usually attend the schools nearest their homes (some areas require a bus ride), attendance at Magnet Schools is usually determined by factors other than geography. Some districts require passing a test of some sort, some require teacher recommendations. Unfortunately, some also respond in some instances to political pressure or favoritism. Still others are operated in order to maintain a specific racial balance.

If your young child attends a Magnet School it is important to maintain the same vigilance and attention as if the child were in the local neighborhood school. It is sometimes very tempting to think that a different school will assure a different program—one that will be better than the norm. Although this sometimes is indeed the case, it certainly isn't guaranteed.

Check out the Magnet School with all of the care you would use investigating a neighborhood school. Take a *walking tour* described in a later section, and ask questions. You may determine that the Magnet School is exactly what your child needs—or you may discover it really isn't any different from the school down the street. If there are any differences, do they make a difference in the educational opportunities, or are the differences only cosmetic? Wherever you look, interview. Interview the teachers, the principal, and other parents. You have the right, the need, and the obligation to find out all you can. Take nothing on face value. Let's look at the other factors to be considered.

Discipline and Academic Performance

In most surveys of schools, discipline—or the lack of discipline—is high on the list of parental concerns.

Generally, discipline, or pupil control, is better in private schools than it is in the public schools, and there are many reasons for this. Private schools can be selective in whom they accept for admission, as well as whom they allow to remain after admission. If children are continually disruptive in a private school, they are removed. If they are disruptive prior to admission, they simply are not admitted in the first place.

The cost of private schools also plays a part in the discipline. If parents are going to pay tuition, they are usually more aware of student behavior, and they are quick to intercede. In most private schools, parochial schools in particular, parents play an ongoing and active role. They keep close contact with the teachers and the administration, and stay well informed on all matters related to curriculum and extracurricular matters. Parents of young children in private schools expect and demand high academic performance, and they usually get it.

Of course the type of private school we are describing here is the one close to home—where students attend during the day and then return home. We are not discussing aspects of residential private schools, boarding schools, or military schools that have very different reasons for existing and which operate on clearly defined standards quite different from nonresidential private schools.

Teacher Credentials

One final word about the private school. Carefully review the credentials of the teachers and the administrators. Unlike the requirements for public schools, there are usually no state requirements for certification that must be met in order to teach in a private school. Legally, teachers are not even required to be college graduates, let alone have any degree of expertise in teaching methodology.

Many people assume that private schools employ only the best, and that private education is always better than public education. It is true that *some* private schools are better than many public schools, and they have worked long and hard to acquire that well-deserved reputation. It isn't possible, however, to complacently take it for granted that private is always better just because it is private.

When you are evaluating schools for your young child, consider the private school, certainly, but evaluate it as carefully as you do the public school. At least with the public school you know that certain basic standards must be met in order to continue operations.

In recent years, many parents have elected to send their children to private schools in increasing numbers because of dissatisfaction with many public schools. This trend seems to be increasing even more rapidly as more and more negative publicity is printed about public schools. Stories are commonplace about public school teachers who can't spell, who write sentences filled with errors, and whose spoken language presents a poor model for young children.

If you come in contact with such inferior teachers, be sure your children do not have to spend any time in their classrooms. You don't have to subject your child to such treatment, and no principal can require you to do so.

Home Schooling

Besides the private school and the public school, there is yet another option that is little known but nevertheless, is used by some. Rather than send their children to any school at all, some parents elect to keep the children at home and teach them themselves. In most states this is perfectly legal.

Check in your state, however, before you decide to embark on this course. There are many variations to this home schooling and to the laws controlling it. Let's focus on some of the major considerations.

First, parents must be capable of providing instruction. This means that parents must not only possess the intellectual ability to help their children learn the material they would learn in school, but sufficient time, energy, and perseverance to accomplish this monumental task.

If there is concern about such things as text books, films, and other media, don't worry. In most instances, the local school is required to provide such material for use at home by parents and their children. In addition, there are further services that local schools provide upon request, such as standardized testing, health screening tests, and diagnostic services.

It is also possible for the student to gain access to the school library, gymnasium, and other related services as well as participate on athletic teams and in other extracurricular activities.

The local school must know of the parent's intent to provide home schooling in advance. The parents can then take advantage of the school's support services and have their child included on the school roles to fulfill the requirement of reporting to the state.

From one perspective the idea of home schooling looks very attractive, especially when we consider all of the previously mentioned services. The truth of the matter, however, is that home schooling is hard work for both the child and the parent. Usually, the parent means the mother. In addition to taking care of a home and a family, preparing, monitoring, and evaluating an educational program at home is time consuming as well as physically and emotionally draining.

If, for whatever reason, you wish to undertake such a task, be sure to contact your local school district early in your planning stages to be sure you can do it in your state. There are some restrictions, and they change from time to time, so it would be inappropriate to give any specific directions here.

Check with your local district. If you don't get a clear cut response, or are not convinced of the validity of the answer, check with the county and state board of education to get their opinion. You should also review the laws governing education in your state. Check the reference section of your public library for a copy of the pertinent statutes, or write your state board of education.

Be prepared to be told "No" when you first ask your local district for permission to teach your child at home. That response often comes for a variety of reasons. Sometimes the person you ask simply does not know the law, and rather than researching the question will simply tell you it cannot be done; that it is illegal. In other instances, school officials are just plain reluctant to give up any control of the education process, so they are predisposed to give a negative response.

Another reason for frequent nonsupport of the request is that because it is rare, school officials conclude it must be illegal, or it would have been done in the past.

Don't take the first "No" for your final answer if you seriously want to offer this option to your young child. The ultimate answer might well be "No," but take your time, and be sure of the validity of the answer in your area before you give up the thought.

I must emphasize again, though, that home schooling is hard work. Don't think about going into it as anything other than hard work. It can be exciting and rewarding for both the parent and child, but you'll *earn* those rewards; they won't come easily.

It's also important to consider the social impact of keeping your child out of the regular classroom that her or his friends attend. The social aspect of development requires social interaction, he or she could suffer some social limitations and emotional handicaps, and in some cases, they can be severe.

A Variety of Options

It is clear you have many options in selecting a school for your young child:

- Public Schools: neighborhood, magnet school, laboratory school
- Private Schools: general, parochial, boarding, military (mentioned, but not described)
- No school: Home schooling.

Whichever you select for your young child remember to consider the following:

- Visit the schools you are considering—often and at different times of the day.
- Talk with the principal, teachers, parents, and other children about their perceptions.
- Determine what you feel is best for your child. Discuss this openly with school personnel to get their opinions.

- Consider keeping your child at home. What would that mean to you? To your child? To her or his playmates? To your other children?

Finally, whatever course of educational action you take, monitor it carefully to determine how it is working. None of these decisions will be "engraved in stone" so you can change your mind at any time. A caution, though. Don't change your mind too often or too quickly. The impression created by such vacillating and indecision can cause young children to become confused and apprehensive about themselves and their abilities. It is up to you to provide order and logic during these early formative years.

Once again, it is easy to see the *partnership* in action. The parent and the school personnel must work together for the benefit of the child. Discussion of options with teachers and administrators, evaluation of progress and educational needs, and discussion of problems and successes as they arise lay the groundwork for success.

Don't delay investigations and discussions of your final choice. Your child deserves prompt, well-informed decisions, and you have so many options from which to select that it would be a shame and a disservice to your child not to explore all of them fully. In the long run, your young children just might want to go to the school where all their friends go and that could be an excellent long-term choice, that should be weighed with the others. The important factor is not to make your decision through indecision. Take the time to acquire all the facts, and then make the decision after a careful analysis.

Picking the "Right" Teacher

The teachers with whom your young children spend their early years can be an inspiration or an impediment to their education in later years. When it's time for a young child to go to school, parents are usually told who the child's teacher will be. No questions asked! "The teacher will be . . ." But, it doesn't have to be that way. Parents deserve a say in the matter, and they will get it if they expect it, ask for it, or perhaps demand it.

In some instances, when a school is very small, options are not always possible. If there is only one first grade or kindergarten, the child's teacher is set. In many instances, however, more than one teacher teaches each grade. When there are multiple sections of grades, parents should voice their preferences about the teacher they feel is best for their child.

What Makes the "Best" Teacher?

What should a parent look for in picking the *right* teacher? *Training, experience, personality,* and *track record* are among the most significant variables, and they are relatively easily defined and observed.

What Training Did the Teacher Have in College?

There has been an ongoing discussion about what subjects a prospective teacher should study before entering the classroom. Some educators suggest that the emphasis be placed on specific subject matter areas, while others believe it is more important for teachers to know "how to teach." They emphasize methodology as the principal area of concentration.

It seems rather obvious that both are needed. It is certainly necessary for a teacher to know how to teach, but it is equally necessary for that teacher to know something about what to teach! Without content, nothing can be taught. That would be like typing without words. You can go through the motions of hitting the keys, but nothing of any sense will be captured on paper. Nothing is communicated. On the other hand mastery of content without the ability and skill to communicate will not lead to the child's intellectual growth and development.

You will want to ask the principal about the training of the teacher into whose care you will be placing your young child. Some questions that may be helpful are the following:

- What college did he or she attend?
- What was her or his major?
- Was it an academic area? Which one?
- Was it "education?" A social science?
- Where did he or she first become certified? In this state or out-of-state?
- What kind of certificate does the teacher have?

Let's expand on these items for a bit. In order for a person to teach in a public school, he or she must meet specific requirements set forth by the state board of education. This means that certain courses must be taken in college, usually consisting of some mixture of academic subjects and educational methods courses.

If you are concerned about specific areas of preparation, you can easily check the individual college or university requirements by getting a copy of the school catalog.

Teaching Certificates

There are many different types of teaching certificates and each one has its own specific requirements. Teachers should be teaching only at the grade level and in the subject areas (where appropriate) for which they are certified by the state. Slight variations exist from state to state, but generally the major types of certificates are as follows.

1. *Early Childhood.* Allows a holder to teach preschool through grade one. The emphasis in training is usually on child growth and development. Motor skill development and social interaction usually contribute greatly to course work.

2. *Primary Certification.* Holder is authorized to teach kindergarten through grade three. Training usually includes growth and development, but it also includes strong emphasis on reading instruction, number facts, and writing skills. The academic component of the training is usually confined to stressing elementary factual material that might be taught in primary grades.

3. *Elementary Certification.* This enables the holder to teach in grades kindergarten through eight. Obviously, this is a much broader certificate than the first two mentioned. Since all of the certificates can be acquired during a typical four-year college period, it is reasonable to assume that a different level of intensity will exist in the training for a broad certificate than for a narrow certificate. For the elementary certificate, prospective teachers will usually study the reading, writing, and basic math areas, but they must also explore science, history,

geography, and other areas that will be covered in the elementary grades.

As for the academic level, it is necessary to point out that the sophistication of these curricula is not as high as it would be if a student were to major in math, science, or history. Teacher education courses are taught on a much lower level.

A generalization: The higher the grade in school, the higher the emphasis will be on subject matter; the lower the grade, the greater the emphasis will be on development and social skills.

That difference in emphasis is—or should be—reflected in the college training of the teacher. Inquiring about the type of certificate, therefore, will provide valuable information in the selection process.

4. *Secondary Certification.* This usually allows the holder to teach in grades seven through twelve. The focus in this certificate is on a specific subject area such as math, science, social studies, reading, English, music, etc. The degree of academic sophistication here is comparable to that of a specific major in one of those academic areas. In fact, some colleges require students to declare an academic major, and their methods courses are in addition to these area requirements.

Because the emphasis in the higher grades is on academic subjects, it stands to reason that the teachers in those areas are expected to take additional coursework in the specific subjects.

Such additional study will provide a sufficiently high mastery level for teachers to lead and challenge the students in the upper grades.

Over all, that distribution looks pretty good, and the varying levels of certification in specific subject areas makes good sense. But, you probably noticed the overlap in the grade levels for which the various certificates apply.

Early Childhood	preschool—grade one
Primary	kindergarten—grade three
Elementary	kindergarten—grade eight
Secondary	grades seven—twelve

It is possible, therefore, for different teachers to be assigned to specific grades yet have quite diverse levels of preparation in the materials that receive attention at those grade levels. A teacher with an elementary certificate, for example, could teach a lower grade level class where reading readiness and reading are most important, or a junior high class where American Literature would be of paramount importance. That's quite a range!

Likewise, secondary certification would enable one to teach physics to advanced students in a high school as well as general science to seventh graders who are just starting to develop the maturity to do simple work in a laboratory. That, too, is quite a range!

When any single certificate covers such a wide range of class levels, it is certainly appropriate—and often advisable—to inquire about the college training and the specific certificate the teacher holds when you are working through the selection process of picking the right teacher. Be sure the level of training matches the emphasis of the grade to which the teacher is assigned.

There are certainly great differences in the specific preparation received from different colleges throughout the country, so simply looking at the grade level and the certificate is not sufficient to give you any absolute answers concerning who is the right teacher for your child. This factor is only part of the information you will need to help make the determination.

Next, you will want to ask about the experience that has been acquired since the initial certificate was awarded.

- How long has the teacher been teaching at this level? At this school?

- What else has the teacher done? This could include curriculum development, teaching at a local college, writing books and articles, speaking to professional associations, and a host of other activities.

- In what kind of continuing education programs has the teacher participated? Study groups? Seminars? Special courses?

- Has the teacher participated in travel and visitation to other schools, states, countries that have broadened the teacher's experiences and knowledge?

The point here is that certification to teach is but one step in preparing for the teaching process. Continuing to learn is essential, so that the teacher can relate to the students as time passes, conditions change, and information expands. Continued growth is essential.

Two very diverse quotes apply here. The first is from *Alice in Wonderland,* "You have to run as fast as you can just to keep up. If you want to get anyplace, you have to run twice as fast." The other is from a school superintendent who hired me for my first teaching job. He said, "I like to hire people who will teach for twenty years—not one year twenty times."

It may help to keep both of these thoughts in mind when you are asking about the teachers who will assume partial responsibility for the education of your young child. Have they been well prepared in the first place, and have they continued to grow and develop so they can assist your child in that same process?

The Person Behind the Certificate

Now, let's look at the person behind the certificate. This is where you must make an important subjective judgment. What kind of person will be best for your child? Disciplinary? Friendly? Supportive? Tough? Intellectual? Creative? Old? Young?

This is a difficult thing to decide objectively because it depends so much on the personality of your child, and to an extent, on your personality. You must consider what type of person elicits various responses from your child. Does he or she need narrow focus and direction, or are broader opportunities more appropriate and effective at this stage?

There are at least two ways to get an idea of the personality of the teacher with whom your child might work. One, of course, is to visit the classrooms where the teachers are conducting classes. What do the teachers do? How do they do it? What kinds of materials do they use? How do they treat their students? How do they talk to them?

Qualities you will want to look for may include warmth, support, and developmental participation; or is there coolness, distance, and tightly controlled direction? Do all of the children seem to be excited and learning? Do they seem genuinely interested in what is going on in the classroom? Is there activity rather than boredom? Do the children share ideas, information, and materials, or is there possessiveness or extreme competitiveness evident throughout the room?

A supportive teacher is a guide and will be aware of the need to develop a strong positive self-image in each child as well as the ability to identify and manipulate letters and numbers. During the classroom interaction this will be evident by the teacher "talking with and to" students rather than "talking at" them.

Some teachers will be seen as firm, and others might seem "laid back." Your responsibility as the parent is to get behind that surface image and form a complete picture. This is where and how we can observe the differences between "teaching" and "learning" as discussed earlier.

Set up a conference with the teachers, ask what they do, and why they do it. Ask them to be as specific as possible in explaining how they get to know each child and about how they encourage each one to actively pursue learning.

Watch out for jargon. Every business and profession has its own vocabulary and members are quick to fall into using it. Jargon can be effective if all parties in the conversation understand what it means, but sometimes it is used to gloss over items and to avoid clear cut responses. If you hear such jargon coming from teachers, don't hesitate to pause and ask for an explanation in plain, simple English. It might slow up the conversation for a few moments, but you'll come out of the meeting better informed than if you try to continue with gaps in your understanding. Teachers should be excellent communicators, but if all parties don't understand the language there won't be complete communication.

Learning Materials

Part of your conversation should deal with references to the materials the teacher uses. Ask about textbooks, for example. Do all students in the class use a basic text, or are many different books used? What are the purposes of each? Is a sample available for you to examine? Does each child get a workbook of some sort or are materials distributed a page at a time? Why? What else does the teacher use? Films, video, records, computers, etc.? Why? When? What materials are the children expected to provide themselves? How will they be used?

Parents are often hesitant to ask such direct questions because they feel a bit out of their element. Don't hesitate for a moment! Be considerate of the teacher's time, make appointments for discussions, and show respect for the teacher's position, in a friendly and positive approach—but get the information you need.

The Teacher's "Track Record"

You're going to turn your young child over to this person for a substantial part of each day, so you should know as much about her or him as possible. You should feel comfortable in turning over your child's time to this teacher. If you're not comfortable, the child will perceive it. That could have both short- and long-term effects on how the child reacts to going to school and learning from this teacher. The best possible outcome of your discussions is the establishment of mutual understanding and the basis for ongoing communication. The worst possible outcome would motivate you to get another teacher for your child. And in the long run that would be good!

Now there is one more important source of information available to you in this selection process. What is the teacher's "track record?" How has this teacher performed in the past? Usually the most direct source of this information is close at hand. All you have to do is ask other parents and children. Talk to parents whose children have been taught by this teacher. There is a tremendous amount of information available just for the asking. "What do you think about. . .?" "How did your child like. . .?" "Tell me about. . . ." Any such comment will open up a flood gate of reactions and information. Certainly, some of it may be exaggerated or biased, some of it might be more emotional than factual, but if you ask enough people you'll get a pretty accurate picture of the teacher and what results he or she gets. Talk to children about the teacher as well, in an open-minded and casual way.

Ultimately you will have examined numerous subjective and objective factors including colleges attended, certification, personality, and the reaction of other parents and children. The sum total of your investigation will certainly enable you to make a rational and informed choice of the best teacher for your child.

One more caution—and piece of encouragement. We all went to school, and we all remember pretty well that the teacher was in charge. Teachers were the ones with the power, and we never felt comfortable or confident in questioning our teacher's decisions about anything. That feeling often carries over into adulthood, and many adults still feel inhibited about questioning a teacher. Don't! Remember that you are another adult who shares the teacher's interest in the success of your child. There is much that is interesting and even fun to share. You may well find that in addition to furthering your child's education you will have made a friend who respects what you are trying to do, and will help you to do it.

And interesting phenomenon has taken place in recent years, and you should be aware of it during this selection period. Now, for the first time in history, teachers are not a great deal better educated than the general population. In the past, many teachers were a select group who had been able to have the rare advantages of higher education. Today, a much larger part of the population has also had that advantage. The teacher of today can expect to work in partnership with a parent population that is far more aware of the goals and methods the teacher works with, and more appreciative of the roles both partners take.

In talking with teachers you are not communicating with a "select, elite" group; you are talking with other people who have a specific job to do and a role to carry out. Carrying out that role requires your cooperation on two levels; one physical, the other emotional.

You must agree to let your child attend the teacher's class, and you must then support that teacher's attempts to help your child. If differences arise you should both expect and agree to air them openly and quickly. Because of what is expected of you, you must know what to expect of the teacher. The education of your young child is, indeed, a *partnership;* and you must know, respond, and trust your partner in order for the process to work. Of course, the teacher has the same responsibility, and the duty to do all in her or his power to instruct and inspire your child, and to work cooperatively with you.

Walking Tour   When you walk around inside a school building, what do you see? There is a big difference between looking at things and seeing something. Very often when we walk through a place with which we are unfamiliar, we find that we look at a great deal, but don't always see what is there. In order to see we need: a frame of reference, a focus, and some specific questions.

So, let's walk through an elementary school and see what we can find.

A school's atmosphere should be conducive to learning. Everything about it should encourage students to gather and use information, skills, principles, and concepts. Learning should be the primary activity.

Because learning is a personal matter, it follows that there should be a great deal of personal attention. Provisions should be made for each and every person to learn what is required and expected of her or him. There should also be opportunities for special, unique activities over and above the basic curriculum program.

In an earlier section we discussed the differences between teaching and learning in relation to schools, but let's review those factors again quickly. If the emphasis in an institution is on *teaching,* then the things that are done, the materials used, and the schedules followed are focused upon the convenience of the teachers. If, on the other hand, the emphasis is on *learning,* then the things that are done, the materials used, and the schedules followed are for the benefit of the learning student. Keep those differences in mind during your *walking tour.* Remember, you want to determine what is going on by being aware of various options.

Waiting or Doing Things

One factor is easily observable by paying attention to what students are doing in classrooms and other instructional areas, like the library and the gym. Ask yourself, "Are they doing something, or are they waiting to do something?"

In some school programs, students spend a great deal of time waiting—waiting until everyone has finished the assignment, waiting for homework to be collected, waiting to go to the blackboard to copy an assignment, waiting until everyone is quiet, waiting for the bell to ring, waiting to shoot a basket, waiting to go to lunch, waiting to check out a book, waiting to go home, etc. Waiting time is usually nonproductive, frustrating, and boring.

It is also a time that can lead to discipline problems if the waiting time is too long. The teacher causes this situation, but the student suffers. When one child is waiting it may mean that some other child is doing something. That other child might be getting the attention of the teacher or some kind of special assistance. That child may be learning something because he or she is active and participating. The waiting child, however, is simply marking time. Because learning requires active participation, waiting fills up the day but not a young, inquisitive mind. If there is too much waiting, the inquisitive mind loses interest.

So, make a mental note about "doing" and "waiting to do." You may see small groups of students working together on a variety of tasks, and this can involve cooperative activity rather than excessive waiting time. In such small groups the children can be assisting each other rather than waiting for a turn. The excessive waiting situation usually develops when the entire class is managed together, as a single large group.

You'll probably also see a variety of activities requiring small group participation. Varied classroom organizational structures require groups of different sizes to work together. Such coordination and small group activity usually enhances the quality and productivity of the time in school. Good teachers can often manage classroom organization well by working with many small groups within the same room. Such organization allows them more time to instruct each child individually, an important factor for each child that emphasizes learning experiences.

Now that we have considered these general comments, let's get on with our walk. As soon as we step inside the building we begin to collect data from which we can form opinions. The first thing we see is the hallway. What might we see?

If children are present there, what are they doing? What are their options? Are they sitting in small clusters reading? Testing each other in various areas of numbers, colors, letters, and the like? Perhaps they are telling stories, or making up songs. Drawing and coloring are often done here in order to complete a bulletin board or a display.

If you see children in the hall, look to see where the teacher is, or if there is a teacher's aide present. If there isn't an adult nearby there could be a problem with lack of direction and control. State laws vary greatly, but there is a nearly universal requirement that a teacher or other responsible adult must be constantly present in a school setting. Aside from the legal requirements, it is sound educational practice for a teacher to be present to guide, direct, and correct students engaged in learning activities. Feedback and direction are important parts of the learning process, and the teacher is there to provide such support. Children, being children, are limited in the extent of the support they can provide for their peers.

Teacher's Aides   We mentioned responsible adults in relation to providing support, direction, and supervision; and such people are important in schools. Teachers have primary responsibility for implementing the curriculum and for guiding the activities of the children, but they need help. Fortunately, in many areas such help is readily available.

As a parent interested in taking charge of your young child's education, ask about the help that teachers receive. (Perhaps you can even provide some assistance.)

Assistance for the teachers comes from a variety of sources. The first is the paid teacher's aide. These people are part of the regular school organization and staff. They are paid by the Board of Education and have specific duties and responsibilities. Their duties are determined in general by the principal to meet the requirements of a particular staff and facility. Although the tasks are varied, they usually include:

- Assisting with classroom instruction in specific subjects such as reading and math
- Helping with field trips
- Helping with art and music programs
- Preparing, securing, and duplicating teaching materials
- Assisting with the supervision of athletic activities
- Taking attendance
- Correcting papers
- Doing research

You will probably notice that in every instance where students are present, the function of the aide is limited to helping and assisting. The aide is not a teacher and cannot—or should not—be expected to provide the services of a teacher. They help, but they do not replace the teacher as the leader of the classroom.

In some large urban school districts teacher aides are, indeed, being placed in teaching situations and are functioning as regular teachers. This happens often in classes where instruction is provided in a language other than English. Some school districts are experiencing difficulty in hiring enough bilingual teachers, and consequently are calling on aides to serve the full role of teachers. It is an inadequate solution (in most cases it is illegal) and it provides less than optimal instruction for the children in those classrooms.

Sources of Teacher Aides

Where do teacher aides come from?

There are a variety of sources, but teacher aides often start out as parents interested in the schooling of their children. They spend time at the school, get to know the faculty and staff, volunteer their services, and when circumstances make it possible, they become employees. Often, those who become aides have had some college level training, which is certainly an advantage because they can anticipate and follow the intent and directions of the classroom teacher.

Sometimes their primary contribution lies in the creative, artistic areas, where they can supplement the talents of the classroom teacher. Although the teacher must provide the direct supervision of the children, teacher aides with such special talent can, indeed, provide instruction in these areas. The teacher must oversee and guide this instruction.

Often, the mothers of young children enrolled in the school become teacher aides because such a position enables them to assist with the education of others, earn some money, and schedule work hours that coincide with those of their own children.

There are many other sources of teacher aides. Senior citizen and retirement homes are excellent sources. Seniors can be a tremendous advantage to schools in general and to kindergartens in particular for at least two reasons. First, those who are interested in such work usually love children, and are very dependable. They can be relied upon to provide support and comfort in a loving, caring way; and they will pay attention to the needs of individual children.

Second, they provide grandparent figures for children. As our society continues to be highly mobile, more and more families become separated by great distances. As a result, it is impossible, or at least impractical, for young children to spend much time with their own grandparents. Children usually need and want a grandparent figure who pays attention and is interested. If circumstances or geography prevent them from having access to their real grandparents, seniors as teacher aides often fill that need.

Children often see the senior citizen teacher aide in a different light than they see their teachers. They often are more readily seen as friends and supporters rather than authority figures. The seniors can often provide tremendous resources and can be called upon for many reasons in addition to the typical tasks mentioned above. such as:

- If they have traveled, they can talk about foreign lands—or their impressions of their travels.

- They can describe jobs they had in earlier years.

- They can describe life as it was many years ago.

- They can talk about games and toys from their own childhoods.

Young children are fascinated by such information, and coming from a teacher aide it seems more interesting and perhaps novel in the school setting. It is *fun*—not *work*. We discussed that difference earlier and here is another very practical example.

Just as the children enjoy being with seniors who are far removed from them in age, they also enjoy working with others who are older than they are, but who are not grandparent figures: they like working with teenagers.

Teenagers can be great with little children! They still remember what it was like when they were little. Helping little ones master all the "hard stuff" of school is fun for many teens, and those who participate in this activity make a substantial contribution to the experiences of little ones.

So, as we continue our walking tour, observe the variety of teacher aides you might pass in the halls as well as in the classrooms. They will be providing a great service by increasing the amount and intensity of personal attention every child receives and needs. They also reduce that "waiting time" we discussed earlier.

Furthermore, although some teacher aides are paid, many are volunteers. This includes all categories: parents, seniors, teens, and others. Because they are volunteers, they are in the schools working with young people because they want to be there. They want to do whatever they can. Certainly, they are getting something out of the experience—a sense of contribution, a feeling of being needed—and that's fine. All educational and social interactions should be two-way streets. All parties should contribute *and* benefit.

Find out from the teachers and the principal how the teacher aides are located, trained, and evaluated. There are many different systems, so it would be difficult and inappropriate to try to describe all of them here, but your local professional educators can explain your particular situation in detail.

Ask them to be specific in their descriptions. After all, it's your child who will be associating with the aides, and you want to be sure you know about their backgrounds, talents, and interests.

Hallway Scenes   Now, back to the halls. What might you see? *Bulletin board displays.* Bulletin boards usually are covered with something, but look to see if you can determine how long the display has been up. In respect to holidays, that's easy. Halloween figures just before Christmas vacation could indicate a lack of interest in providing appropriate holiday theme displays. That could also indicate other factors, e.g., no time during which the teacher, an aide, or a student could prepare such a display. That's possible, of course, but it's highly unlikely. Neglect could also indicate too little money for supplies. More and more this has become a practical reality. No imagination might explain the deficiency, though that is highly unlikely since the media and the public press, as well as professional journals, are filled with suggestions and ideas, and teachers usually take advantage of them. Perhaps, no one cares. This could be the case, and if that is so a real problem exists.

If you see displays that are obviously outdated be sure to ask the teachers, principal, and children why. Some bulletin boards are not so obviously out-of-date, but it's easy to determine how long displays have been up. Just move an element of the display—a letter, drawing, or a figure—and see if there's a mark on the bulletin board surface. Just as pictures that hang on a wall at home leave a mark, after a time, bulletin boards record such long lasting displays clearly.

Individual teachers are usually responsible for the displays adjacent to their classrooms. You might also ask them how they use bulletin boards at the school. Are they decorations? Are they to serve some educational purpose?

Look for announcements on bulletin boards. These are usually found near the main office. What is being emphasized? Meetings? Policies? Schedules and other similar administrative data, or educational items such as seminars, lectures, and courses? There will probably be some of both kinds. Let's hope so, anyway. Try to determine what receives emphasis.

Such emphasis can tell you a great deal about the focus of the school in general, and it's a good clue in determining if this is a good place for your young child. If the emphasis is on administrative duties, the school could be staid and rigid, but if the emphasis is on growth, then the programs could be flexible and conducive to learning. This alone, of course, will not be sufficient data upon which to form a firm conclusion, but it can help.

Finally, there is one more thing that can be found in the halls which can be a strong indicator of what to expect throughout the building and the program: graffiti! Graffiti is interesting not only for what it says, but the fact that it is there in the first place.

Graffiti on walls, restrooms, furniture, or materials indicates lack of respect, a lack of pride in the physical surroundings. If there is much of it, it reflects lack of pride on the part of the students, but also indicates a lack of pride on the part of the adults in the building— the principal, the teachers, and the others who have direct professional responsibilities there.

If graffiti is tolerated, what else is tolerated? Be sure to observe and ask questions.

Classrooms

So much for the hallways for now. Let's start looking at classrooms. The first question to ask yourself is how crowded is the room? How many children are in each classroom? How many teachers and teacher aides are assigned to each room?

Size

There is wide-ranging research on the optimum class size at various grades, but educational research, like other social science research, is sometime inconclusive and even contradictory. No one has yet been able to state with precision and certainty just exactly what number constitutes the absolute best size for a class of students. There is pretty general agreement, however, that somewhere between 25 and 30 students per classroom is a maximum-sized group. If the class size begins to get much larger, problems develop related to individualized instruction, discipline, and academic advancement.

There isn't the same concern as the class size becomes smaller, however, because there is even more chance for individualized attention; and, of course, taken to the extreme, a small class can result in nearly private tutoring. Although that might be fine for academic skill development, it may leave a great deal to be desired in relation to the development of social skills.

So count heads, both large and small. One teacher for 25 students is a reasonable ratio. If there happens also to be a teacher aide, you're in luck. Most likely, though, the teacher aide will be found only in classes considerably larger than 30—if at all.

Next, look at the sizes of the students to see if there is any marked difference. Ask the teacher or other responsible adult if the class is a single grade or multiple-grade. In other words, are all the children about the same age and in the same grade, or does the group represent two or three grades and a correspondingly wider age range?

Age Range

There is varied thought about the acceptable age range for children in grammar school. Some educators are convinced that a narrow age range in a single grade is the best way to provide educational opportunities. Others feel that since age is only one variable in the development of a child it should not be the primary factor in selecting an organizational pattern. They feel it is better to have a wider age range in a single classroom with that range encompassing two or three grade levels. In that way material can be covered and opportunities provided when they are appropriate for the students, rather than when a more fixed curriculum guide indicates they are to be presented. Some of the names for this arrangement are Open Primary, or Integrated Primary, etc.

Such multi-age, multi-grade organizational patterns require additional work for the teacher, but many factors indicate that the growth of the students is enhanced because they can learn and explore at their own rate rather than at some externally controlled rate.

Some parents become concerned when they think their very young children will be placed in classes where they will have to compete with older children. That competition factor is the culprit. In multi-age groups, children have the opportunity to move fast if they are able to do so and to move more slowly than their classmates if they have that need. The pace of academic and social growth can easily fit the pace of physical and emotional development if the schools elect to concentrate on that area. If two or three years can be spent in the same classroom setting, the instruction can be more fully individualized.

When there is multi-age grouping there will often, but not always, be a teacher aide or a regular volunteer to assist in the administration and instruction of this more complex group.

The instruction and complexity relate directly to the use of time that we mentioned earlier. As you observe the class in action pay attention to what individuals are doing. Although the class as a whole will be doing things, that class is made up of many individuals, and you should focus on how each child is actively spending her or his time in the room. Are the children involved and participating—at all times—or at least most of the time—or are they waiting for their time to come? Are they doing things or are they looking? Are they active or passive? Are they "waiting" or are they "doing?"

Learning requires participation, not just observation.

Participation can be enhanced by a teacher who is comfortable and competent with multi-age groups. Ask your principal and the perspective classroom teachers what they think of such grouping. Be sure to ask them to explain and justify their responses; don't let them simply say they agree or disagree with the concept. Your questions will ensure thoughtful answers. If you don't get them, watch out for that school and that teacher. If teachers can't justify and explain what they are doing, perhaps they don't know what they are doing!

It is not my intent to push for multi-age groups in favor of single grade organization, but it is appropriate to state why I have made repeated references to this type of structure. Simply stated it is because most people think of schools in terms of single grades. Since that is the case, and since most people are familiar with the benefits—real or perceived—of single level classes, there is no need to detail them here. On the other hand it is appropriate to point out some of the varied factors related to multi-age groups in classrooms because they are unfamiliar.

It is necessary for each and every parent to assess the impact of the class composition. The chances are excellent that the child will have no difficulty whatsoever, if the teacher is good, and comfortable with this arrangement. This is a rather safe statement to make since the children have already spent most of their preschool lives in a multi-age environment; their families, neighborhoods, and religious groups are all multi-age; and the children have already developed many social skills with these groups.

Organization   It is interesting that school is one of the few places that is so organized on the basis of age. Furthermore, that age limitation applies only to the students. Teachers, principals, and other adults are not grouped by age. The question naturally arises: why must children be grouped in this way? Adults are organized on the basis of experience, ability, and potential; why shouldn't children be organized on those bases, too?

Ask the teachers and the principal to explain why the classes are organized as they are. Ask them to be specific. If they do not yet have multi-age groupings, and you feel it would be helpful, ask about the possibility of this option.

Regardless of whether the classes are organized on the basis of single age or multi-age, look for another factor in the structure of the school. Find out how many different sections there are of each grade and/or of each multiple-age group. In other words, how many kindergartens are there, how many first grades, second grades, etc. This information can be very important to you and your child in the future.

As with any social interaction, personalities come into play in schools. Sometimes a student and a teacher don't like each other. Oh, they try to get along, often barely making it, but they make it. But, they just don't like each other. If such a personality conflict poses a problem, or better yet, before it becomes a problem, you will feel much better if you have the option to transfer your child to another section—to another classroom.

Wherever there are multiple sections of a grade the chances of affecting a good match between child and teacher are increased. If there is only one place to put a child, he or she is faced with a set of problems that could otherwise be avoided. Of course, such multiple sections are not always possible. School enrollment might not warrant it. In fact there are many schools across the country where just the opposite is true. The total school enrollment is low enough to require that children of various ages be placed in the same classroom.

The one-room school house is the ultimate extension of this situation, and many well-educated, well-prepared adults have received their early education in the one-room school. All of the various arrangements can work well if the teachers are good and comfortable with the structure.

As you continue on the walking tour, keep track of your options. You might have to take the initiative in discussing the most appropriate placement of your young child when the time comes.

You know your child better than anyone else does, and you have the responsibility to share appropriate information with the school personnel. Sometimes the school personnel won't ask for it, but you should feel free to provide it anyway. The actions of the school will be based on what they know, so help them to know about your young child.

If the school people happen to reach a placement conclusion different from yours, for example, that's understandable; but be sure to push for—and get—a clear explanation and justification for their decisions. If they can't provide that, don't agree with the placement. In a partnership all partners are equal and have an equal say. Partners are also entitled to share in the bases for all key decisions.

Sometimes educators will try to sway you to their position with a sentence that begins like this: "Based upon my experience, it is my professional opinion that . . ." Ask them to do better than that for justification. You have experience based on first hand contact with your child that can direct your parental opinion. It is certainly as good as the educator's opinion, so further discussion and investigation are clearly in order.

Now, let's continue on the walking tour and look at some other elements that make up this thing called school.

The Library

Let's look at the library. The first question to ask is, "Is there a library in this school?"

If not, where must students go for additional information to supplement what they get in their classrooms? Is there an easily accessible public library? Are the students left to their own devices? Must the parents provide all supplementary material?

If there is a library, let's take a look at what it has to offer and at what it provides on a daily basis.

First of all, find out how the children get to use it. Ask the following questions:

- Can they go there on their own?
- Must they go at a certain time?
- Is going to the library required?
- What can they do when they get there?

- Can they do free reading? Read anything?
- What help will they get in selecting material?
- Is there a librarian there at all times?
- Is the librarian trained and certified?
- Will other students be able—and expected—to help?
- Is it a quiet place?
- Is it just one big room with many tables?
- Are there any separate study/work rooms?
- What evidence is there of work in progress? displays? projects?
- Are there any materials on special display?
- Who develops such displays?
- How long do they stay up?
- Are there any themes in evidence? Seasons, authors, or types of literature?
- Are the students encouraged to be active?
- Must they sit and be quiet?
- Can students come and go to the library on their own with permission from the teacher, or must whole classes go to the library together?
- Is student work displayed? What kind? How often? How long?

Materials Look to see what kinds of materials are housed here. Are there only books and other printed material, or does the collection include films, slides, records, video, and pictures?

The reason for this short series of questions is to provide a chance to look at what we can expect to find in many libraries today.

Not too long ago, the library's primary function was housing books and other printed material. It was a print-oriented, print-dominated facility. The furniture was designed to be used with print material. The librarian knew all there was to know about collecting, storing, and distributing printed material. Print was seen as the primary method of providing all information. All that was needed to furnish a library was tables, chairs, shelves, a card catalog, and a charge desk.

Then came the information explosion, and with it came a variety of media in addition to print. There were heated battles about which medium was best, which was good, and which was bad.

Slowly, films, records, slides, filmstrips, television, and computers became part of the library collection. It was difficult for many people to call a place where such a collection of nonprint items was housed a library, so a new designation was created. Media centers, resource centers, and instructional material centers began to appear. That was where all the nonprint material was kept.

Facilities

Initially, there were separate facilities, separate rooms, separate personnel. The library housed the books and the librarian, the resource/media/instructional materials center housed everything else and the media specialist. There was overlap and duplication, and there was clearly a turf battle.

In most cases now the turf battle is over, and a negotiated peace has been accepted.

The word library has remained, but the collection housed there has changed. So have the furnishings, the floor plans, and the personnel.

Today, you can expect—in fact you *should* expect—to find a variety of material housed and readily available in the library (resource center). Print and nonprint, books, video cassettes, slides, films, computer programs, cassette tapes, records, and picture collections now all receive equal consideration.

Tables have relinquished some space to listening carrels—those small, three-sided booths that provide semiprivacy for viewing projected material and listening to audio materials through headsets, so as not to disturb the quiet environment.

Computers are likewise available; some for use by patrons and others to supplement the tried-and-true card catalog.

Workrooms have been added wherever possible, and their presence, along with the carrel and the varied materials have brought on the current situation where self-instruction is possible through the use of a variety of materials.

That has created an opportunity for students with a limited interest and/or ability in reading to gain access to relevant study material. Further, material is not limited to what can be printed on paper; now the instructional medium is determined by the content to be covered. Some material is most appropriately covered by the printed book, but other material cries out to be presented in sound with motion and color.

In many respects the library, both the school library and the public library, has become a kind of information supermarket. Various materials are on the shelf side by side. It's no longer necessary to go to two or three places to find material on a desired topic. Everything is cataloged in one place, and a single search will yield listings on books, magazines, motion pictures, audio tapes, etc. There is ease of access to the listings and to the material itself.

So, look at the library (resource center if the name hasn't changed yet).

- What is there?
- What are the students doing there?
- What are the adults doing?
- Is there equal access to a variety of media?

If you can't get the answers through your observation, ask. Ask the children, the librarian, and be sure to ask the principal. If the library is the same as it was years ago—only books—ask for reasons why.

As with the other elements in the walking tour, in order to get an accurate picture, you'll have to take the library tour more than once. Plan to visit when the students are present as a complete class and individually. Visit when there are no students so you can talk with the librarian, who would otherwise be occupied. Watch as the librarian presents information to individuals and to whole classes when the teachers are present, and when the teachers leave the classes under the supervision of the librarian.

Interestingly enough, the tone of activity you observe in relation to the library will often reflect the tone of the entire school. Excited inquiry, active participation, and academic support here will also be found in classrooms. If the library is a rigid, quiet, controlled, overly-orderly place then the classrooms will probably be much the same.

A visit to the library might just be an opportunity to view a microcosm of the entire school. Your observations there can help put other items into perspective. Of course, this is a generalization, and you are cautioned to investigate the school fully. The impression gotten from the library is an important part, but it's only that—a part.

Physical Facilities

So far we have been concentrating on the intellectual and social parts of the school observable on this walking tour. Let's now look at what we can find out about the physical elements and programs as represented by the school gymnasium. Once again, a simple question: Is there a gym?

If not, ask the principal about the physical education program—if one exists.

- Where do the children learn sports?
- Where do they get help in developing coordination?
- Where do they learn games and skills?
- How is their physical growth and development tested and recorded?
- Where do they learn sportsmanship?
- Is an organization other than the school responsible for these activities?
- If so, which one(s)?

If there is a gym, what should you look for? First of all, is there a gym teacher? Is there a physical education specialist available to determine and provide for the physical needs of each child?

Physical differences in young children are perhaps more widely varied than any other differences, and the perception and skills of one specially trained in this area are very important.

Next, what kind of equipment is available?

- Is it in good repair?
- Does the extent and variety of the equipment match the needs of the children?

- Is there a planned program for the entire year to reflect and provide for growth and development, as well as seasonal changes?
- Are there records kept in view to encourage students to perform to their potential, rather than to just emphasize competition?
- Is the environment clean and conducive to participation?
- Is total physical well-being or only performance emphasized?
- Is there a variety of activities offered to accommodate the interests and abilities of all the students?
- What kind of competitive sports program is there?
- Is the program separate for boys and girls, or is it coed?

In addition, look at the relationship between the physical education teacher and the classroom teachers. Do they seem to regard each other as "colleagues" or do they see the presence of the other as "time for a break in the routine?"

- Is it cooperative?
- Does the classroom teacher drop off the class and disappear until the gym period is over?
- What assistance and advice does the gym teacher provide to the classroom teachers and to the principal?

If there is no physical education teacher, what does the classroom teacher do to provide instruction in this important area? Some classroom teachers are quite good with games and sports activities, but physical education is a special set of skills. Ask the principal what you can expect for your child on a daily or weekly basis.

While we're looking at physical activity, let's walk over to the playground to see what's there. The playground serves a variety of functions.

It's a place for children to burn off energy before entering the school building.

It's a place to develop sportsmanship and skills under the watchful eye of the teacher. It's a place to develop social skills with peers. But for our purposes let's be a little more specific.

- What size is it in relation to the size of the student body?
- Can all of the students play here at the same time?
- Is it clean?
- How much grass is there?
- What facilities are included? Baseball, volleyball, soccer, other?
- What equipment is there? Swings, jungle gym, slides, other?
- What kind of supervision is evident?
- Are there always adults present when children are present?
- Is the play all free play or is it organized?
- What kind of protection is there from traffic? from unwanted visitors? from strangers?
- What kinds of rules apply? Rough games? Snow balls (where appropriate)? "Big kids"/"little kids" areas?

Since the playground is visible to everyone passing the school, its conditions and what happens there often influence how people perceive the entire school program. This could be true for you also.

You will probably be familiar with the outside of the school and the grounds long before you start the walking tour of the entire facility. It is easy and tempting to form an opinion on the basis of what is outside, on the basis of what can be seen walking past the building, or on the basis of what others tell you they saw.

Because it's so easy, we held off the visit to the playground until after we explored the rest of the building and saw some of the program elements that are readily observable. Every one of the items we examined is an important aspect of the total school program. The playground is as vital as the others.

We skipped a couple of obvious places like the principal's office, health room, and teachers' lounge; they don't have the same impact on the educational offerings as the other areas we looked at. Of course it's important to look at their general condition, cleanliness, and accessibility, but they are not the places where the children will spend most of their time and which will greatly influence their behavior or progress. Indirectly, of course, these places can affect the children because their teachers will have spent a part of their day in those rooms, but that's not a major consideration for you during your tour.

You should, however, feel free to visit them just to see if they reflect the rest of the building facilities. There should be no startling differences in the quality of the furnishings and the state of repair between these facilities and the classrooms, libraries, and the other widely used areas. They should all measure up to an acceptable, appropriate standard.

The entire facility, needless to say, should be kept in repair, clean, and safe. Such physical conditions will enhance the possibility and probability of learning although they cannot guarantee that learning will take place. What the faculty does within the physical surroundings, and the manner in which the faculty employs the materials at their disposal will have the most profound influence on your child. What you do to learn about the school and its programs, its strengths, and its shortcomings will enable you to work with the faculty to establish conditions conducive for your young child's growth and development.

The partnership will pay off, and this walking tour will help you to understand the factors which create the conditions of the partnership better. Happy walking!! And, as they say in the stores: if you don't see what you want—ask!!!

The Special Role of Kindergarten

During the walking tour, you should make a special effort to visit and talk with the kindergarten teacher(s). Because of the great variation in child care and preschool programs, it often falls to the kindergarten teacher to evaluate the progress of the child's education thus far, and to provide the instruction and educational program to help fill in the gaps, to be sure the child is ready for first grade.

Readiness, especially in reading, mathematics, and social development, is measured formally and informally in kindergarten, and you will want to be on a mutually trusting and communicative basis with the kindergarten teacher. There is much that you can do to make sure that you are informed on your child's progress, and to take part in her or his progress yourself. If there are special educational needs, you will be all the more involved.

Even if your child is not yet at kindergarten age, visit the kindergarten teacher(s) on your walking tour, introduce yourself, and make it clear that you would welcome a talk, when it is convenient. You can build up a good relationship with the teacher your child will have, long before he or she is in the kindergarten group. If your child is closer to four or five, and kindergarten is imminent, set up an appointment as soon as possible.

At this point, ask the teacher to describe the kindergarten program, and to let you borrow curriculum materials to review.

Make sure that you understand the curriculum, and ask the teacher to point out how it relates to the first grade program in the school. Be sure to be considerate of the teacher's time, and plan ahead so that you and the teacher can meet without time pressures hanging over your heads.

As with all teachers, you will want to be sure to express your appreciation of the demands the teacher must meet. Be sure that you are considerate of these, while you see that your own needs for your child's education are met.

If you can establish a good relationship, and demonstrate your willingness to cooperate and your ability to take part in your child's education, you will have prepared the way for a productive kindergarten year. On this basis, you will be able to meet any problems that arise with better communication and the means to discuss and resolve them.

Understanding of the curriculum, and how it relates to first grade will be helpful.

This "understanding" doesn't have to be a deep intellectual activity. Simply ask the teacher, "What do you do?," "Why?," "How?," and "How do you know it works?"

In other sections of this book we have used the word "specific." It certainly fits here. When you ask questions of the teachers *be specific*. And expect specific answers.

All too often teachers (like most other professionals) like to talk in generalities and in jargon. Don't settle for such responses to your questions. You can't assess a general statement and its impact on your child's future; you must *know* what an answer means.

It's the teachers job to present the clear answer. You shouldn't have to figure out what the teacher meant! You should have it made clear to you. You provide the question—the teacher provides the answer.

Jargon is verbal shorthand. It isn't always intended to evade or confuse, but often it does! If you became aware of the use of jargon, stop the flow and ask for clarification. If you don't understand the meaning of the words you can't be an equal partner in the conversation. When that happens there is not communication. When you ask for clarification, and demand it, you'll be able to judge the accuracy of the answer.

It will also give you an opportunity to evaluate what is to be learned, and decide if there are additional needs you feel should be met. If there are other needs, you can choose to discuss them with the teacher, and urge their inclusion in the activities. As an alternative, you can plan supplemental activities of your own. If there are serious problems, you will want to get additional advice. One good source is the nearest college department of education, or the state department of education. The resource person may advise you to speak up firmly, to approach the principal, to confer again with the teacher, or none of the above. You will have to weigh the advice you receive, and make your own decision; but you will be better informed about the situation than before, and it will make your decision easier.

It is certainly just as likely that you will find very positive situations in the kindergarten, and find that you and your child simply enjoy the school activities all the more when you know the curriculum, the teachers, and the school, and can take part readily in the progress of your child's kindergarten year.

Primary Grades

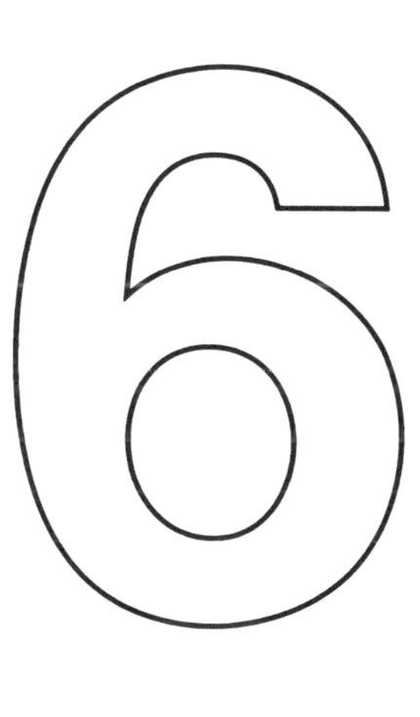

First Grade and Beyond

For many children, the beginning of first grade is the beginning of "real school." At least in their imaginations, and in the descriptions of their friends and perhaps older brothers and sisters, first grade is often looked upon as a far more serious undertaking than earlier forms of school.

For parents, too, the beginning of first grade represents a somewhat more serious concern. It brings with it an additional set of questions, and the desire to understand what can be expected of the school. What will it contribute to their young child's education?

The walking tour offers opportunities to familiarize the family with the physical plant, the special facilities, and the school's personnel. For the young child, it provides an important orientation that can allow the child to feel much more comfortable when the actual first day of school arrives. Knowing where the child's classroom will be, whether the first grade is a part of an upgraded primary grouping that will include second and third graders, whether the child will have teacher or a team of teachers, are all important factors.

The parent will also want to be familiar with the organization of the school's staff, and to be familiar with the personnel, and their particular areas of authority and responsibility.

The Principal: What Can You Expect?

The official role often designated for the principal is "Educational Leader." That's what it should be, and leading the total educational program of the school is how he or she should devote her or his time and efforts. We'll talk about what that means in just a bit, but first let's discuss what he or she often must do rather than what he or she should do.

There is a great deal of "administrivia" required of a school principal, including:

- Supervising the ordering and distribution of supplies.
- Securing the services of substitute teachers on a daily basis.
- Coordinating school bus pick ups and deliveries.
- Writing reports for the central office.
- Filing out forms for the research department.
- Scheduling room use for a variety of teacher, parent, and student organizations.
- Administering small budget allocations for special projects and student activities.
- Investigating discipline problems.
- Monitoring custodial services and performance.

These are just some of the many and ongoing activities that must be carried out by the school principal. Without attention to such details the instructional program would certainly suffer. They, in effect, provide a foundation on which the instructional program rests. Like the foundation of a building, these are out of sight, unseen by the casual observer, but if they are not solid, in time the entire structure will crumble.

The specific tasks will vary, of course, from school to school, depending on such factors as size and availability of assistants. The tasks, however, must be carried out by someone.

Now, let's look at the instructional leader and see what that means to you and your young child. What should the leader do?

The principal should assure that your child is always placed in the most appropriate classroom setting, with the most appropriate teacher in order to foster a desire for life-long learning through success in acquiring basic skills, and developing concepts and principles.

That's a long way of saying the principal should do everything possible to help your child learn all he or she can!

How does that happen? What should you look for? First, of all, determine if the principal is accessible. Call up, and ask to schedule a meeting to discuss your child's entry into the school—or your child's program if he or she is already in school. Can you schedule the meeting in the immediate future, or must you wait? If you have to wait, find out why. Is there a backlog of appointments with other parents, or is the principal buried with that "administrivia?"

You can also get a feeling for the principal's accessibility during the walking tour of the building. Where is the principal? Before you can walk around most schools you will be required to sign in at the main office, so you'll find out immediately if the principal is in the office. Is he or she there, or is he or she walking the halls and visiting classes?

Some principals choose to run their schools from their offices, requiring that teachers, students, and information come to her or him there. Others, however, spend a great deal of time in other parts of the building, collecting information first hand.

Certainly, some of both types of activity is necessary in most cases, but see if you can determine the extent to which your principal spends time in each place.

As you try to get a picture of the principal and understand what he or she does, ask a few questions such as:

- Does the principal visit classes and watch teachers teach?

- Does he or she meet with individual teachers to discuss how well they are doing—or where they need to improve?

- Does the principal teach classes personally? On a regular basis? A regular subject? Once in a great while?

- Does the principal participate in extracurricular activities? Coach a sport? Direct plays?

- How does he or she relate to the students in general? Is the principal liked, respected, or feared?

- What do the teachers think about her or him? Is the principal liked, respected, or feared?

- What about the feeling of parents toward the principal? Is the person seen as an advocate or as a judge? Does the principal know the students—by name?

Perhaps this last question is the most important one to ask. Being the instructional leader doesn't mean administering a large enterprise; it means providing guidance, direction, and support for each and every child in the school. If the principal doesn't know the names of the children in the school, what assurances are there that he or she is able to provide individual attention?

Some principals feel that the classroom teachers are the ones most responsible for assuring this individual attention. Although there is some truth to that it is certainly reasonable to expect the principal to at least know who the children are that populate the building, isn't it?

When you send your child to school, don't you expect the principal to know who this little person is? If you call or visit to inquire about your child's progress, won't you expect recognition? Of course you will. So determine if the principal knows the names of the children in the school. The principal has a responsibility to guide their development, so he or she should know them. During the years your child attends school you should expect that the principal knows her or him or there is little hope or expectation the principal will help in the child's development. And that's the principal's primary job! That's what an "educational leader" does!

Let's assume for a moment that your child is just starting school. You want to know in which classroom, and with which teacher your child will be placed.

First of all, set up a meeting to discuss this major event in your child's life. It is not a major event in the principal's life so you must take the initiative. If you don't arrange a meeting, your child's name will be put on a class list on the basis of such factors as birth date, sex, and total number of students. In all fairness the principal will probably have little other information about your child at this time.

But you know everything about your child!

So arrange for an opportunity to share your knowledge with the principal before a class assignment is made. The earlier the better, because the structuring of a class of young students can be a complicated process, and the more available information there is for each child the better the grouping will be.

Sometimes individual principals will request to meet with parents of incoming children, but don't take the chance that this will happen. Call, and assure it will happen.

When you meet, be open with the principal, and tell him or her what kind of child you will be sending to school. Ask what he or she and the teachers will do with, to, and for your child. Use the following questions as guidelines for the meeting.

- To what teacher will your child be assigned? Why?
- What will happen if the assignment turns out to be an inappropriate one?
- Can the child be switched to another classroom?
- What effect could such a move have?
- Whose decision will it be to move the child? Yours? The principal's? The teacher's?
- If you think the teacher isn't right for your child what can you do?
- If the principal determines that a placement is not good, what is done? When and how will you find out?
- How does the principal monitor how well the students are doing in order to consider the need for a change?
- What information does he or she get from teachers on the progress of each child? Does it come routinely? Sporadically? Only in an emergency?

- Does he or she meet regularly with teachers to discuss progress and needs?
- What about discipline? What happens if a child fights? Steals? Cheats?
- What is the official policy on discipline?
- What variations and modifications might be expected?

In addition to such specific questions, you should inquire about the general operation of the school program. We all know about grade levels—kindergartens, first, second, third grade, etc., that children are assigned to such levels primarily on the basis of age, and that their activities are pretty well defined.

But what else is there?

What Other Services and Professional Supports Are Available?

Ask the principal to describe the total program in the school—and in the district if some services are provided that way. Ask about the availability of professionals, in addition to the classroom teachers, in such specialties as:

- Speech
- Music/band
- Art
- Drama

Are there professionals in:

- Library services
- Learning resources
- Social work
- Psychology
- Learning disabilities

What services are available for special education?

- Physically handicapped
- Emotionally handicapped

- Socially handicapped

- Home hospital care

If such services are available, ask for specifics such as:

- How many are available in each category?
- How often do they meet with students?
- At what grade levels are they available?
- What kind of coordination is there with the classroom teacher?

If there are teacher aides in the school, ask about them.

- How are they selected?
- What are their qualifications?
- Do they ever teach children without a teacher present? (Watch this one very carefully. The answer should be "No." That's the law, but all too often, especially in crowded urban schools, aides do teach—without the direct control of certified teachers. In schools with a high incidence of non-English speaking students, teachers are sometimes difficult to find, so aides do the teaching.)

If you think your child might require some special education consideration to assure her or his successful growth and development, tell the principal, and ask about the process used to identify the needs and prescribe the program.

He or she will probably describe a process often referred to as a "staffing." This means that the principal will call together specific professionals and charge them with collecting pertinent information that will be used for the benefit of the child. A staffing usually includes the classroom teacher, a psychologist, a social worker, some special teachers (music, art, etc.), and, of course, the principal.

Together, this group shares and evaluates the information each one presents from her or his unique perspective, and then prescribe the specific action to be taken.

This might include: classroom placement, therapy, special classes, additional psychological testing and counseling, and/or other appropriate action.

The group then meets with the parents to explain their plan in detail and will report periodically to the parents. Certainly, this can be one of the most significant activities for a child in order to assure that maximum learning will take place during her or his time in school. The staffing is a specific activity and it is obvious when it takes place.

The role of the principal, as instructional leader, should assure that similar attention is paid to each and every child in the school. Not every child requires the specific and focused attention of a staffing, but each child needs and deserves this type of support.

The instructional leader must assure that this happens.

He or she must be accessible to the parents, to the teachers, and to the students. The principal must have first-hand information about the educational activities of her or his school through observation, evaluation, participation, and contribution.

The principal must assure that the system operates smoothly and that the business and "administrivia" are taken care of, but only so that a firm foundation will support the entire learning environment.

As a parent you have the right to expect such support and activity. You have the responsibility to work with the educators so that, together, you can provide the learning environment your child needs.

Once again, we're looking at a *partnership*.

Teachers: What Can You Expect from Them?

There is an almost infinite variety of answers from which to choose. Of all the areas we have explored so far, this is perhaps the most difficult because there are so many kinds of teachers: young—old, new—experienced, male—female, traditional—experimental, flexible—rigid, creative—mechanical, competent—incompetent, etc.

If we take the teaching profession as a whole and try to answer the question, "What can you expect from them?" The only logical answer is, "almost anything!" That, however, is not a reasonable answer and it certainly won't provide any direction in searching for ways to assure the best possible educational opportunities for your child.

Rather than trying to respond to "what can you expect" let's focus instead on what you *should* expect from a teacher into whose care you place your child.

Although it is almost impossible to precisely rank a listing of qualifications, perhaps the top ones would include the following:

- Communication ability
- Knowledge
- Inspiration
- Empathy

Of course we could include other factors to lengthen the list, but we would probably find ourselves identifying a variety of subsets rather than adding new specific subjects. What should you expect to find under these categories?

Communication ability: the business of teaching is the exchange of ideas. The focus is on helping young children to acquire facts and skills, and then apply them in the formation of new principles and concepts.

You should expect teachers to:

- Establish environments that encourage and permit learning,
- Use materials that match the interests and abilities of their students,
- Apply strategies that encourage students to learn—and to enjoy learning,
- Continue to learn themselves in order to relate to their students as time passes,
- Share information with you!

The classroom environment should be stimulating, interesting, clean, and safe. Physical characteristics are important in a classroom. Children cannot be expected to learn or to want to learn if they don't feel safe and comfortable.

When children enter a school, they expect to find things to learn and ways to learn them. Teachers therefore, have both the opportunity and the responsibility to provide stimulation to an initially receptive audience. If teachers present the stimulation, the response is continually learning and interested students. If the stimulation is removed or is minimal, interest declines.

We sometimes speak of the natural curiosity of children, and although much curiosity exists in their early years, if children don't see rewards from that curiosity, it soon goes away.

As we said in an earlier section, before they enter school, children see learning as fun and exciting. After they start school, learning often becomes hard work. When that happens the children don't want to do it anymore.

Who causes the attitude change?

Interesting situations and opportunities produce interested people. Look around your child's school. Is it an interesting place to be? Would you like to spend six to eight hours there every day?

Teachers are the ones who create or destroy an interesting environment.

What Are the Teachers in Your Child's School Doing?

There is yet another area in which you can observe the communication ability of teachers. When you visit the classrooms and walk the halls, pay attention to the materials the teachers have prepared. Also, when your child brings work home containing comments by the teacher, or announcements from the teacher to parents, read them carefully. Pay particular attention to spelling and grammar.

You might be very surprised—even shocked—at what you find. As the *best and brightest* college students have moved from schools of education to other schools, the verbal skills of many future teachers have declined. Today more teachers with poor communications skills exist than did a generation ago. Be aware, and be concerned about this development. If some of your teachers have not mastered the basic skills, how can they help your child to do so? Some teachers might not even know where errors exist, much less how to correct them!

Be particularly aware of what materials teachers use in their classrooms. Do the materials reflect the present world of the student or the past world of the adult? Is that classroom environment filled with only printed material, or is there evidence of other media? We are not suggesting that every classroom be a multimedia showplace in continuous performance, but we are suggesting that the exciting and involving world outside the classroom should be reflected inside the classroom. Certainly, the expectations of the curriculum must be met, but there are many ways to respond to any challenge or opportunity.

If the emphasis in the classroom is on learning, as we have explained, then the material used should be appropriate for the learner. It has often been said that schools are for the children, not for the adults, therefore, what is used should be appropriate for the learners. In applying basic learning or communication theory, it is essential to begin identifying the characteristics of the audience. Only when communicators know the composition of the audience can they design and transmit effective messages.

Teachers can accomplish these instructional tasks with ever-changing student bodies only if they themselves understand that changes are taking place. Teachers should constantly add to their understanding of the world and the children's view of that world. It is the responsibility of teachers to know what makes the students function. It should not be the responsibility of the students to figure out the teachers and what they want.

And now, the final communication function: sharing information with you. This, too, is part of the teacher's responsibility. As a parent, you have every right to expect a continuing flow of information from teachers about your child. You should expect to be called for periodic conferences throughout the school year; you should expect to receive regular written reports about your child and his progress. If you don't get such calls from the teacher, make them yourself.

As we said earlier, watch for spelling and grammar. Mistakes may not be important in and of themselves, but consistent errors may indicate significant lack of skills or lack of attention on the part of the teacher. You may want to discuss this, if it is recurrent. If you do, try to be tactful and objective in your comments.

In addition to written communication, you should expect a periodic phone call and perhaps a home visit. The latter is often difficult, sometimes impractical, and perhaps impossible. If visitations can be scheduled, fine. If not, there will always be the *Open House* and *Back to School Night* when you can visit the teachers. Plan to go to these as often as possible. The personal contact will help you and the teacher as well as your child.

Are the Teachers Well-Educated?	*Knowledge* is the second qualification on our list of what you should expect in teachers. They should have strong backgrounds in all of the areas that make for a

well-educated person. Humanities, science, and the social sciences should all be part of the training of the professional adult. Likewise, there should be firm grounding in educational philosophy and history, as well as a clear understanding of psychology and teaching methodology.

Both academics and methods must be present in the education and training of classroom teachers or they won't be able to help your child learn. Academics and methods are both important. One without the other will produce incomplete results.

Recently, changes, many of them very frenetic, have been introduced into the curriculum offerings of teacher training institutions. Many educators have stated loudly that the system is not as poor as a variety of separate reports have painted it to be. The fact that so many changes are being introduced, however, leads one to the conclusion that there have been problems.

If the system had been so good in the past, why should it be changed by adding so many new components? Further, it has been interesting to see how many schools have been given awards of excellence once they adopted some of these hastily developed changes. Many have defended such actions by indicating that it is necessary to demonstrate a positive response to such pressures from federal and state agencies to avoid further difficulties. We must then inquire about integrity and the true value and performance of the local schools and institutions of higher learning.

Evidence seems to indicate clearly that many of the best and brightest college students are, indeed, entering professions other than teaching. In addition, practicing teachers are leaving the profession in ever increasing numbers. If those two factors continue, there will be even greater reason to be concerned and interested in the level of knowledge teachers carry with them into their classrooms.

Inspiration and the excitement of learning and helping others to learn is the next qualification you should expect to see in teachers. They should indicate through their actions that they really want to be in school working with young people.

It should be easy for you to see if they seek out ways to make learning interesting and exciting. Students should catch the spirit of learning from their teachers and carry it with them long after they have completed their formal schooling. If their teachers have that spirit, the students will probably get it too. If the teachers don't have it, however, it is highly unlikely that the children will ever get it.

Finally, *empathy* will enable teachers to feel for their students. It will help them to focus clearly on the learning process and not on the teaching process. Teachers who have empathy for their students remember what it was like to be in school, to struggle with new concepts and skills, to take examinations, and to do homework every night. The teachers who remember are the ones who will be remembered. Empathy makes it easier for teachers to do what is necessary to inspire their students. With it, teachers organize their knowledge of subject matter in a way their students are able to understand and grasp.

So, what should you expect from teachers?

Simply stated, you should expect performance that will make children want to learn, enable them to learn, and encourage them to keep learning.

Those teachers are the ones my former superintendent would have liked. They are the ones who would teach for twenty years—not one year twenty times.

A tall order—but what wonderful results!

What about Parent Organizations?

In the vernacular of the computer age, parents of school children represent a specific "user group." Members of user groups share one common drive: to share information. That should be the primary purpose of parent organizations, too.

Let's look for a moment at user groups. Some are very structured, but many are not. Some are local in nature; others are very general in scope. Some concentrate on specific material; others look at long-range implications.

Members volunteer information on successes and failures with specific material, equipment, and programs. They request assistance from fellow members in solving problems. They test and evaluate products, openly communicate with other members, and provide feedback to publishers, producers, and manufacturers.

These are all voluntary services. Members belong and contribute because they realize they can benefit personally, as well as contribute to the benefits of others.

There is a realization and a demonstration of the belief that freely shared information will be of value to all members. Those with more experience will help those with just a little, and newcomers sometimes bring a freshness and an enthusiasm that encourage even greater investigation and cooperation within the group. They ask questions and raise issues that others might not see because of the changing perspective brought on by the passing of time.

In the user group there is a recognition that diversity of background, experience, and operations focus the applications and uses of the specific hardware and software that brought the group together in the first place.

It is the hardware and software that is the common element; all other factors demonstrate the diversity of the group.

So it is—or should be—with parent user groups. The single common element, of course, is that all the members have children. But, then the differences appear. Some parents have many years of experience with children in school, while others are brand new at this. The experienced ones have already had the opportunity to try out some of the specific of the system—the teachers, and principal, for example; they are in an excellent position to provide evaluation of those elements.

They can describe in detail the successes and failures they have had with each teacher and with the principal.

The newcomers to the parent groups know when, where, and how they can get information to solve their problems relating to those same teachers and principals, to the placement of their children, and to the general practices that govern the school.

There is only a limited amount of printed material available to parents describing the practices and policies of the school district. The parent organization, however, is a constant source of updated material.

Now, some school personnel might argue that much of that material will be biased, reflecting a specific and limited point of view. The same things, however, can be said about the material produced by the school district offices. As interested parents, you should seek out and acquire information from as many sources as possible—then form your own opinions and conclusions.

"Product testing" by the user groups is an ongoing process. Children of members are in constant contact with the teachers so new information about them is always being placed into the system. Free and open sharing of such information gives all members the opportunity to update their evaluations.

Perhaps the "feedback" area is the one that provides the greatest benefit to all members, and to the supplier as well.

It is one thing for a parent organization or user group to collect information and to share it with the other members. Going to only that extent, however, focuses on "what is" rather than on taking steps to influence "what might be."

User groups provide feedback to producers and manufacturers to help them evaluate existing products, and more importantly, to develop and produce new and better products. User groups are important to the producers and manufacturers because they are the ultimate judges of the products.

When there is cooperation through communication between the user and the producer, changes and modifications can be made in a timely, orderly, and productive manner. If the users simply stop buying, the company is out of business and might not even know why it got into trouble in the first place.

So it should be with parent organizations. They must provide feedback to the school personnel concerning the perceived quality of their efforts and results. Parents pay for the services of the schools, and provide their children to the schools as "raw material." Without the children, there would be no schools. Parents should, therefore, feel free to communicate their evaluations and expect the schools to respond in a spirit of cooperation.

If the schools are not responsive, the parents' ultimate reaction can be the withdrawal of their children. When that happens, the schools are out of business.

At the present time, by the way, that is exactly what is happening in many large, urban districts. Because the public schools are unresponsive and not providing what many parents want and expect, parents are sending their children to private schools. If that trend continues, it could mean even greater problems for the public schools in the near future.

Finally, the user group is effective because it is the combined voice of the many members. Therefore, it has power. Parent organizations, likewise, have power, because they are the voice of many parents.

The requests or demands of a single individual rarely get the same response as a group gets in any situation, and that is as true of a school system as it is of a computer company.

Group pressure simply means group influence. As parents, you need influence because you are interested in assuring that your young children are exposed to the best possible learning opportunities available to them.

So look at, and join with, the appropriate parent groups available to you. For those who have not yet had this opportunity, let me list the types. There will be classroom parent groups, schoolwide parent-teacher organizations, and district groups. Of course, there is also the state Parent-Teacher Association and the National Association of Parents and Teachers. They are all worthy of consideration and membership and, they provide a valuable forum for mutual understanding.

As a general rule, the larger the base of the organization, the more general its goals; keep that in mind as you contemplate membership. A classroom group will focus its attention on what a particular teacher is doing, for example, but the National Association of Parents and Teachers will address broad issues such as promoting legislation and suggesting alternatives for providing adequate school funding across the country.

All are important, but you can't give all of them an equal level of attention. So select where you will concentrate your efforts.

First choice usually includes that classroom group and the school group, and that is true for preschool parents, as well as for public and private school parents.

Participation in such parental organizations is a good strong start toward developing that partnership that is so important in directing your young child's learning experiences. You should, therefore, become a member of that users group as soon as you can.

An early start will assure a long-term, productive relationship with other parents as well as with the teachers and principal to whom you entrust your child.

Partners: You, Your Child, and the School

We all get to go through it just once, so we have to make it good. In a very real sense, parents and schools are truly partners. They concentrate their efforts on just one product—children. Parents form the children who are eventually sent to school. Teachers then have the opportunity and responsibility to excite, enhance, inform, and inspire their minds, encourage them to grow strong bodies, and become responsible members of society. There isn't, however, such a clear cut division of labor. Both parties must cooperate or the child may become fragmented.

In the past, tasks were sharply divided. Parents raised children; teachers taught children. The division was clear and understood by all because the teachers were well-educated themselves. They became teachers because they were well-educated. Children were sent to schools to learn, and it was assumed that parents were not able to provide what teachers could.

As time passed, however, those differences have disappeared. In fact, as we stated in earlier sections, today a very large portion of the general population is as well-educated—or better educated—as the teachers.

In many areas teachers are no longer viewed with the same respect they once enjoyed. Part of the reason might be a decline in the standards of the teacher training institutions. Part of it might be the result of an attitude shift on the part of the teachers themselves, caused by increased demands of bureaucracies, large classrooms, higher student mobility, and many changes in methods, materials, paperwork, public expectations and workloads.

Now, what does all of this have to do with a statement on partnership? Simple.

Partners must communicate; they must share ideas; and they must recognize that they have a major responsibility for the outcome of their joint efforts.

All through this book, we have said over and over again "ask and tell." Ask questions of principals and teachers, and tell them what you know about your child.

Contrary to all reasonable explanations, there is still a gap between many teachers and parents. Parents often are uncomfortable when they have to talk to teachers.

Teachers are often defensive when faced with parents' questions or dissatisfaction.

That tension—anxiety—increases when parents have to meet with the principal, and it is almost overpowering for some parents to meet with the superintendent of schools. That shouldn't be the case, but it often is.

Now, let's look at the other side—the teacher's. In the past, teachers often called parents to school to discuss the progress or behavior of a child. Parents came, and the teachers were in control. The teachers knew they had a strong position and that, in many instances, they intimidated the parents. Some teachers used that feeling unfairly, in order to maintain control over the situation.

Today, teachers often are hesitant to call parents to school. When parents do come, it is the teacher who feels intimidated by the parents. In some cases the reason for this feeling is the teacher's knowledge that the parents are as well-educated, or better educated, than the teacher.

So we have the makings of a very interesting situation. Parents are still uncomfortable talking to teachers, and teachers are uncomfortable talking to parents. This often results in situations where teachers don't volunteer information, suggestions, or actions to parents; and parents hesitate to ask teachers for information, suggestions, and actions. This situation is too costly to be allowed to continue.

Somebody must break this cycle of silence and hesitation.

While the adults remain hesitant to confront each other, and begin the open communication in such situations, the children are continuing to grow. Time passes even though ideas don't.

It has often been said that we get only one try at life. If we don't do it right the first time, that's it. Unlike the making of a movie or a television production, there is no second take when a scene is not acted out well. In life there is only one take.

Children are the responsibility of adults, and they rely on adults. They will follow where adults lead for many years and will mimic their actions.

When they see that their parents and teachers are hesitant, reserved, and uncommunicative they may reach the logical conclusion that that is how they should act. What they see will be much more significant to them than what we adults tell them.

Parents should provide good models for their children to follow. One of the best ways to do this is to show your children that you are truly interested in their school activities. Help with the work, smooth the way when assignments are rough, and encourage them to explore.

As for your relationship with your partners—the teachers and the principal—open the communication lines as far as they will go. Take the initiative! Ask questions and volunteer information. Start right away—even before your child enters school—because there is no time to waste.

Think again of the analogy we used at the beginning of the book. When we stand on a riverbank and look at the water, we are aware of movement but often forget that a particular drop of water that was in front of us a moment ago is now far downstream. It will never come back to that spot in front of us again.

Because children are moving quickly, adults must be sure their movement is guided, protected, and productive.

A partnership makes that possible.

This Is It! 7

We've come close to the end of our exploration of taking charge and planning for your young child's education. We have discussed learning opportunities that can be provided at home before the child enters any kind of formal school organizations. We discussed the wide variety that leads to different formal school organizations, and we have looked at the qualifications of the people who work in them. We walked through a school and examined a broad range of elements and expectations, and opportunities for opening communications between parents and school personnel.

We are at the point where we must say, "This is it!" We have talked long enough; it's time to get on with the action.

Your young child won't be young for very long. What you do now will affect your child's entire life. It is time to think, plan, and *act* on your child's education. The word *education* itself deals with action. *Education* comes from two Latin words. *E* means *out,* and *ducere* means *to lead, draw forward* or *bring.* So, education suggests both *action* and *direction.* It calls for us to lead out, to draw out. The word describes a very dynamic process!

Many years ago, the great American poet Robert Frost wrote "The Road Not Taken" which, initially, describes a simple decision about which of two paths to take during a walk in the woods. As the poem's theme develops, we see that the entire nature of decision-making, action, and the consequences of action are embodied in the lines. "Two roads diverged in a wood, and I—I took the one less traveled by," writes Frost. Take action now that will affect both you and your young child. At the conclusion of the poem, Frost tells us that he made a distinct choice, ". . . and that has made all the difference."

Research, Think, Choose, Act

The choices you make, too, about your young child's education will make all the difference. The most costly mistake would be not to choose—to remain passive in relation to your child's education.

So, this is it. Research, think, choose, act. Act in concert with your partners—your child and the school, to make the most of the opportunities ahead of your young child in the years to come.

The Rest of Your Job

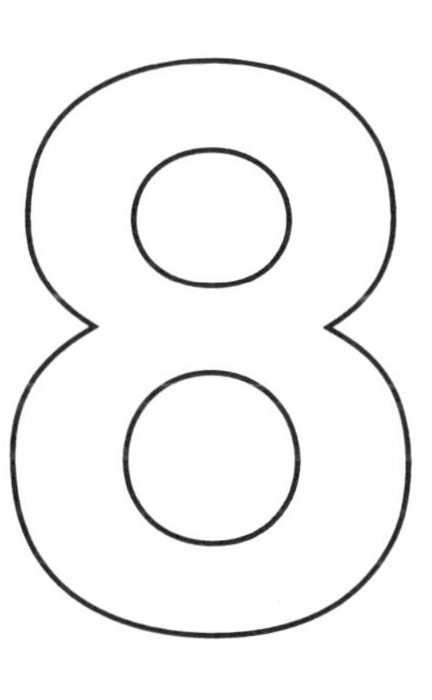

A Brief Statement
We've covered a great many details in these pages, and now let's revisit some of the major ideas.

The responsibility for your young child's education is yours. Schools and teachers will help with the delivery systems necessary to reach your goals, but you have to set the destination.

Your agenda and the school's agenda are different. Look at some of the differences.

Your Agenda	School's Agenda
This is *your* child.	Your child is one of *many*.
Protect and enlighten	Control
Expand the world	Keep things running smoothly
Make learning exciting	Keep the class "together"

There is much more, of course, but the differences are clear. That isn't said to be critical of the education system, it's just an observation, a statement of fact. Someone other than you will not—cannot—know or care as much for your child as you do. Right?

Modeling Behaviors

The process of education takes a part of your every day with your child. Education doesn't start with school. It starts with your child's first breath.

That new "blank slate" that came into the world begins to acquire and process information immediately. And you are the primary source of that information. Everything you do and say has a lasting impact—everything creates an impression.

What you do, for example, will influence what your child will do. If you read, so will your child. If you sit and watch a lot of television, so will your child.

The way you model behavior will be played back by your child in the years to come.

Setting Guidelines

Now here is another idea to work with. Many parents—particularly those who are parents for the first time—feel it is important to allow the child to explore the world with few restrictions. The parent's fear is that the child's "natural curiosity" will be stilted if he or she is told "no." We often hear the comment that the child should be "free to fail." That sounds good in some circles, but if you abdicate your responsibility to lead and direct, you won't be doing your child any favors. The child's behavior will be random. The child has no compass yet. The child doesn't know what the destination is. That's your job. You are the guide—you should not be the follower!

You can assist your child to experience the true wonder of learning if you set up the appropriate conditions every day. What can you do every day? Try these ideas and then add your own.

Talking and Listening

Every day at mealtime talk about what happened during the day. Even before the child can participate, if he or she sees the adults talking that will be the norm when the participation *is* possible.

Ask the child questions—and then listen to the answers. All too often adults don't listen. Listening, however, is essential if there is to be conversation and discussion. These activities are two-way streets. So help your child learn how to navigate on that street. Show him or her how to do it safely. Help your child take risks, but take them safely under controlled conditions.

Make every trip an adventure. The trip might be to the supermarket, but for a young child a supermarket can be a wondrous place filled with ideas and, yes, temptations. But every idea and temptation is a valuable experience and an opportunity for you to help your child to make decisions, suggestions, and requests. That's what communication is all about.

That give-and-take at mealtime or at the store will contribute to your child's feeling that he or she has good ideas that deserve to be shared. The child will learn that communication is fun, rewarding, and helpful. The child will also learn that he or she is good at it.

We all know when we feel we are "good" at something we'll do it over and over. We'll enjoy it. The same is true for your child. *Help your young child to be good at learning.*

Help yourself to get good at it too by trying some of these ideas starting right now.

You don't have to wait until your child is getting near school age. Your job starts right away. You can't wait. Your child certainly won't wait to start learning. The only question is, what lessons will be learned?

Making Decisions

As we said in the first chapter, you must decide what you want. And you should write it down so it's very clear. If you can't write it, you won't do it.

You can't put off this activity. It has to be done starting on day one, because that's when the learning starts. You can't allow for "trial and error" because you can't "rewind" the tape and try again. When time passes, it's gone! But that pressure can also heighten the excitement of learning. If you make learning an adventure to be shared by everyone in the family it will live with your child until long after the "young" days are over.

So that's the rest of your job.

You must take charge. That means you must know about the process and the activity, and you must be active. You can't take charge if you don't participate.

Your job is to set the course and to set up the proper conditions. The professional educators will assist later with the implementation, but you must select the destination.

This takes work, and it takes commitment, but the results are worth the effort.

Good luck.

Additional Sources of Information: Associations and Organizations

The following is a selected list of associations and organizations that specialize in educational interests, and in the interests of parents, teachers, and administrators who share the responsibility of educational programs. They are dedicated to the development of communication, and the dissemination of information on educational practices, theory, method, policy, and law. Many are specifically oriented toward helping parents maintain an active role in their children's educations.

For information, address the Director of Public Information or the President. It is helpful to enclose a stamped, self-addressed envelope to facilitate replies.

American Education Association
P.O. Box 463
Center Moriches, NY 19934

American Montessori Society
150 Fifth Avenue
New York, NY 10011

Association for Childhood Education International
11141 Georgia Avenue, Suite 200
Wheaton, MD 20902

Council for Exceptional Children
1920 Association Drive
Reston, VA 22091

Division for Physically Handicapped
Hopper Education Center
1101 Bay Avenue
Sanford, FL 32771

EPIE Institute (Educational Products Information
   Exchange)
P.O. Box 839
Water Mill, NY 11976

Foundation for Gifted and Creative Children
395 Diamond Hill Road
Warwick, RI 02886

Gifted Advocacy Information Network
225 W. Orchid Lane
Phoenix, AZ 85021

Home and School Institute
Special Projects Office
1201 16th Street, N.W.
Washington, DC 20036

Human Resources Center
I.U. Willetts Road
Albertson, NY 11507

Institute for Development of Educational Activities
259 Regency Ridge
Dayton, OH 45459

Microcomputer Education Application Network
256 N. Washington Street
Falls Church, VA 22046

National Association for the Education of Young
  Children
1834 Connecticut Ave., N.W.
Washington, DC 20009

National Association of Private Schools for Exceptional
  Children
2021 K Street, N.W., Suite 315
Washington, DC 20006

National Congress of Parents and Teachers (PTA)
700 N. Rush Street
Chicago, IL 60611

National Head Start Association
1707 15th Street E.
Bradenton, FL 33508

National Committee for Citizens in Education
Wilde Lake Village Suite 410
Columbia, MD 21044

Parent Cooperative Preschools International
P.O. Box 15604
Phoenix, AZ 85060

Play School Association
19 W. 44th Street
New York, NY 10036

Prime Time School Television
212 W. Superior
Chicago, IL 60610

Research and Demonstration Center for the Education
of Handicapped Children and Youth
Box 89
Teachers College
Columbia University
New York, NY 10027

Additional special interest associations and organizations can be found in the following publication, which is available in most major libraries: *Encyclopedia of Associations,* Gale Research Company: Detroit, Michigan.

New editions of this two-volume reference source are published on a regular basis, and new and very specifically-focussed organizations appear in each new edition. It may be helpful to check this reference for additional sources of information that may apply to your specific situation, especially if your child's educational needs are unusual in any way.

Guidelines and Additional Sources of Information on Interactive Programs

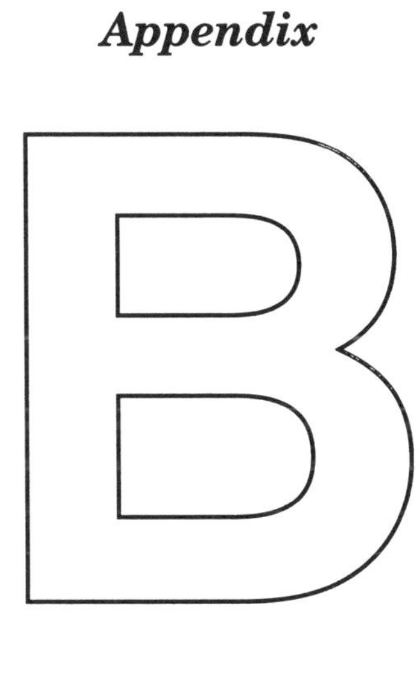

Guidelines on Interactive Programs

As you begin to review material for possible purchase, you will become aware that a great deal of the material on the market falls into two categories: "page-turners" and "drill-and-practice," or "skill-and-drill."

One of the reasons for this is economic: it is easier and less costly to produce such material than it is to develop more complex material that takes full advantage of the capabilities and power of the computer.

Computers available today have the capability of .very complex programs, which can respond with great flexibility to a variety of responses from the users. A program that takes full advantage of this capability is referred to as *interactive*.

Interactive programs provide for truly individualized instruction for the user. What the child already knows will affect not only what information and activities the computer presents, but in what order. Interactive programs make good use of the capabilities of the computer, and provide choices and interrelated continuities that interact with the child's choices at each step along the way. Such programs are difficult to develop, and costly to produce; but they are worth the extra expense in most cases, in the increased learning opportunities they offer your child.

Let's examine the concept of interactive material so you can assess its value and determine the advantages it can offer over page-turners and drill-and-practice materials.

Current literature contains an increasing number of references to the term interactive. In many instances these references focus on the capabilities of machines—the hardware. There are interactive microcomputers; interactive videos; and the current ultimate, interactive personal computers with a video interface. These terms sound impressive, but in truth, it is not the machinery that is interactive because the hardware is doing nothing more than processing information when and how it is directed to do so by the programs. The hardware must have the capacity to provide the breadth of choices needed by the program, but the hardware does not provide the content of the choices at all.

The interactive aspect then is a property of the content of the material, the software. Because most of us are still somewhat unfamiliar with this type of material, it is appropriate to explore how interaction takes place. It is necessary to grasp the basic concept of interaction in order to identify it in existing material you might purchase for your child.

To begin it is necessary to accept the concept that *it is ideas that are exchanged in any interactive relationship.* Such an exchange of ideas requires *application and manipulation of symbols* (words, numbers, signs, etc.). These symbols can be stored in various devices, for later recall. If they are stored in such a way that they can be used in an *orderly and alternating transmission and reception of ideas* by users, they are being used in an *interactive* program.

A simple illustration can help at this point. Visualize two people engaging in a conversation. Party "A" speaks while Party "B" listens. When "A" finishes, "B" speaks, and "A" listens. What each one says in turn depends on what has just been said by the other participant. If that is not the case, then there is chaos rather than interactive conversation.

Each speaker serves as a stimulus for the other. The extent of the interaction and its complexity depend upon the intellects of both parties and their abilities to manipulate the available symbols.

Interactive exchange, therefore, is a method whereby one intellect communicates with another intellect. The contribution of one determines the contribution of the other, and the process must build upon what has gone before.

Let us look at another example. In Situation "A" you tell a friend to meet you someplace—for example at the corner of State Street and Lake Street. The friend responds, "Okay." End of communication. Your directions will be followed.

This is simple direction—no interaction was required. Your transmission of the message could have taken place in person, over the phone, in a letter, or have been relayed by a third party.

For purposes of analysis, the intellectual exchange went *one way only*.

You were in control. You selected your message, your symbols, your time. What you friend thought, said, or did in no way influenced your choices.

Now look at Situation "B" in which the conditions are quite different. When you tell your friend to meet you at State and Lake Streets, the friend asks, "How do I get there?" Then an interaction begins.

You must identify what your friend already knows in order to give effective directions. You must consider:

Does the friend know where he or she is now?

Does the friend know the transportation options available?

Does he or she know the schedules?

Has the person taken similar trips before?

Were the trips successful, or did the person have difficulty?

Will the friend know when he or she arrives?

There are many more questions, but these will serve to make the point. It is only on the basis of the information your friend provides that you can give precise directions. You must ask questions, and the specific answers the friend gives will dictate what specific information you provide, and in what sequence.

You can begin and continue the sequence only after you have received information. If you do not consider the friend's responses, the results of the communication would be unclear, confusing, and wasteful.

In Situation "A" you simply assumed that a great deal of information was already available to your friend and expected the person to gather what was needed in whatever way he or she could. In Situation "B" you provided multiple opportunities for the friend to get what was needed from you.

In Situation "A" you didn't have to know any more than where you wanted the friend to go. In Situation "B" you needed to know not only where you wanted the friend to go, but also how to get there from wherever the person was at the time you spoke. You needed a great deal more information at your disposal. You also needed the ability to question, and to receive, understand, and interpret the information coming from your friend.

In every sense, what you said influenced what your friend said; what that person said influenced what you said; and on, and on, in sequential steps. Certainly, the interactive nature of this exchange can be easily seen. It is truly intellect-to-intellect. The symbols used could be spoken words or written words. They could be delivered face-to-face, via telephone, fax, or in a variety of other ways including, of course, the computer. In this developmental exchange, you would be performing much in the same way as an interactive computer program, and your friend would be performing in much the same way as the *user* of an interactive computer program.

It is clear from this analogy that the *method* of transmission is not nearly as important as the *content* of the transmission at each step along the way.

Interactive programs, therefore, require a large, flexible body of knowledge that can be accessed and manipulated easily, and made *responsive to changing conditions and requirements*. Interactive material requires the capability to react, not just act. Selection and transmission of information are modified depending upon the ability and requirements of the receiver—not upon a rigid structure of requirements from the sender. This, again, is the difference in focus between "learning" and "teaching."

Design of Programs   In the design of such material, at least two major considerations are necessary. *First,* the specific body of material to be covered must be understood fully by the designers and the one initiating the activity. *Second,* provision must be made to identify specific characteristics of the receiver of the transmission. Provisions must be made for flexibility as well as accuracy. If your young child is to use the program, you want to be sure that the child's particular abilities and limitations have been considered and that provisions have been made for the child to build upon the knowledge he or she now has.

If there were to be but one receiver of a particular program, that would not be difficult since the specific characteristics could easily be identified through conversation and observation of the potential receiver. In an instructional program, however, there will be many different receivers. Without a large potential group of users no product would be commercially viable; so it would never get to the marketplace for you to examine.

The program producer, therefore, must make provisions for the specific characteristics of a wide variety of potential learners. A broad range of assumptions must be developed which will accommodate and relate to all of the learners in general as well as to each specific individual. Clearly, such planning is complex, time-consuming, and costly; but it is essential if the teaching–learning process is to be successful.

In order to assure such success, the process often is undertaken in what might seem to be reverse order. It is the application of this process, however, that leads to material that will be of greatest value to your young child.

Sequence of Programs

In the sequence of interactive computer programs the producer should address the following items in this general order:

1. What is the desired final outcome of the lesson?

2. What should the learner know or be able to do *after completing* the lesson?

3. What does the learner know *at the start* of the lesson?

4. What sequence of events/activities will be most appropriate for the learner?

5. How will the learner's progress be monitored and assessed?

In designing the learning activity in the sequence suggested above it is easy to see that Items 1 and 2 can and must be clearly stated by the instructor prior to contact with the learner. Item 3, however, by definition, requires close contact with the learner, and Item 4 depends upon outcomes of Item 3.

It is at these points that interactive material recognizes the abilities of the learner as an individual with a unique set of experiences. The knowledge already present in the learner will dictate the manner, the method, and the techniques that will maximize learning. This technique applies the principles of tutorial instruction at its best, so the opportunity to provide such individualized instruction is very desirable. If the lesson were being designed for a single, known individual the instructional design task could be undertaken with a single prestructured learning path.

Because interactive instruction is intended to address the unique characteristics of any number of unknown individuals, it is necessary for the instructor, the instructional designer, or the producer to assume a wide and extensive set of *possible alternatives* to provide for the needs of the individuals who will work through the lesson. Each learner is unique and will, therefore, follow a specific path through the activity. The lesson must be flexible enough to accept and respond to the individual requirements of each of these possible paths. The instructor must constantly monitor each learner's acquisition of information in order to lead this particular user forward through the appropriate steps which will assure the final mastery of the material.

The Learning Activity

The learning activity is one of ongoing communication—interaction—between the instructor and the learner. What the instructor knows about the learner will determine where the learning path will begin. As the learner demonstrates what he or she knows—at each step—the instructor selects alternatives to lead to the conclusion of the lesson.

Since the lesson is designed in advance of its use, the instructor must assume and plan for as many of the learner choices as possible. This, of course, could be an infinite number, but the realities of time and costs will dictate the actual, final number. The larger the number of interactive choices incorporated in the initial design, the greater the possibility of an accurate and appropriate fit with the unique characteristics of the learning needs of your child.

It is clear that, in interactive communications, the emphasis is on "learning" rather than on "teaching." We discussed these differences in another section, but perhaps a brief recap is in order. If the emphasis is on "teaching" then what is said and done and the material and sequences used are determined by and are for the convenience of the teacher. If, on the other hand, the emphasis is on "learning" then what is said and done and the materials and sequences that are used are for the benefit of the student.

Learning is an individual activity. Regardless of how many people learn from a lesson the acquisition of information is personal and individual. The instructor of an interactive system must, therefore, provide the potential for individual and personal experience.

Finally, the storage and transmission techniques are only methods by which two intellects communicate—the learner and the instructor. The technological state of the art will determine the physical carrier of the information, but both the program content and the user involved will determine the success of the transfer of information.

It should be remembered that there is a valid use for noninteractive materials, and if the needs you wish to address are for practice and drill, certainly there are excellent materials for those uses. It is necessary, however, to be able to tell the difference, and to be able to choose on an informed basis.

Computer-Related Sources

Computer technology is changing so rapidly that it is necessary to develop a sound foundation of information on how they work and what they will do, in order to make decisions concerning purchase and use. Earlier, we made a brief overview of the basic facts. It is suggested, however, that you also review some of the print material available to help you decide what will be best for you and for your young child.

Books

Most of the major bookstores today have extensive collections of computer-related material. Visit these bookstores—as well as your local computer store—and just browse! There is plenty to look at and to try out.

Journals   Subscribing to a computer journal will give you ongoing information, and provide you with more advanced information on computer programs, and their uses, both for educational purposes and other home uses. Subscription prices vary, as do the frequency of the issues.

You should write to the journals that interest you, to request subscription information. You may want to examine copies of the journals in your local library, to see which ones may fit your specific needs best. Since new journals are being published at a rapid rate, your library may be able to offer many additional choices, as well.

In addition to the library, you should visit your local bookstore. The larger bookstores carry an incredible variety of books, magazines, and journals on computers. Most stores now have entire sections just for computers and for educational material to use with them.

In fact, a few recent visits to both libraries and bookstores convinced me that the stores often are much better stocked than the libraries. That's partly due to the selection acquisition process. As soon as materials are published they are in the stores. Libraries, however, must go through the purchasing process, which slows up the delivery.

You'll also see that the personnel in the stores are often more familiar with the computer material because they specialize in that area. Library personnel have responsibilities for numerous areas.

Visit both. Have your questions ready. Take your time in making decisions. Make your own list of materials that will be of value to you and to your young child.

Your list will be much better for your young child than any I could draw up. After all, it's *your* child!

Kindergarten Curriculum Areas

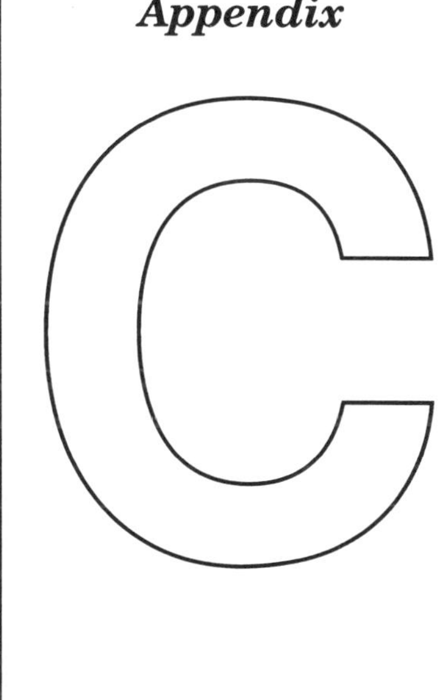

The kindergarten curriculum has evolved during the last two decades to a degree that was unheard of in previous school eras. Many progressive educators in the earlier parts of the century conceived of many of the most important curriculum areas and some developed activities and learning sequences in some famous classes for a time. But it is in the last twenty years in the United States that early childhood and kindergarten learning has received a great deal of attention, hard work, and importantly enough—funding from all levels of government, and many private groups.

Today we have much information available, and many well-developed programs at the kindergarten level. This is not to say that our knowledge cannot be improved, of course. It is only to say that the curriculum that has been developed is a good and useful one, rich in many of its aspects, and a great advance over the less-formed concepts that guided us in most cases, such a short time ago.

A brief list follows, as a sample of areas in the kindergarten curriculum. Be aware that different terms, emphases, and lists are used in many, many places. The list that follows is to serve as a *general description only*. You will be able to consider some of the basic areas of concern, the skills involved, and some general levels of development that are the goals of learning activities in kindergarten.

Try to bear in mind that this is not an absolute list any more than the curriculum guide you may receive from your school could be either interpreted or applied as an absolute—it is a general guide, and as such it will help you to familiarize yourself with some of the terms and structures used. Don't be surprised, or upset, however, if it doesn't conform exactly to another curriculum guide your school uses. This in itself is no cause for alarm, and is to be expected. That having been said, you will no doubt see many familiar areas, and terms also, when you review your school's curriculum guide; and this list will have served its purpose to that end.

Motor and Psychological Development

Many of the children's achievements depend on a physical and psychological readiness, and the following gives a general list of areas that can be expected to have developed by kindergarten level, and perhaps long before in most children.

1. Gross motor development—the child can crawl, run, hop, jump, and skip, and can throw a ball, kick a ball, follow a line walking, hop or jump into squares or circles in floor games.

2. Fine motor development—the child can hold pencils and crayons, draw simple shapes, hold paint brushes, and use plastic or clay molding materials. Eye-hand coordination and small muscle coordination is developed during the year, and the child will be able to make distinct shapes in letters and numerals, and draw human figures and other familiar shapes.

3. Individual, small-group, and large-group activity— the child will be able to share in small- and large-group activities, of short duration, share toys and

materials in games (also for short durations), and play individually with creative materials. These activities will be varied, and the child will be given opportunity for interaction and for individual activity.

4. Sensory and perceptual development—the child will be given opportunity for development of visual, auditory, and other sensory activities, and will be able to distinguish by sight, sound, touch, odor, and temperature in games and other activities.

Memory of sensory experiences and use of names and other symbols will be developed.

Language Skills

1. Description—children will observe and describe colors, sounds, shape, sizes, textures, temperatures, and other physical properties in games and activities. Concepts and terms of comparison, classifying, categorizing, interpreting and drawing conclusions, and sequencing will be included in activities.

2. Vocabulary—names of the basic colors, sounds, shape, size, texture, temperature, including:

Red, orange, yellow, green, blue, purple, brown, black, white, and a variety of shades and hues. Loud, soft, whistle, song, toot, thump, rattle, bang, ding-dong, tap, hum, bark, meow, others. Round, square, triangle, circle, ball, cube, tube, rectangle, oval, oblong, others.

Large, big, small, little, tiny, huge, medium, middle-sized, and comparative and superlative forms, others.

Soft, rough, lumpy, smooth, slippery, scratchy, sticky, others.

Hot, cold, warm, cool, burning, shivery, chilly, others.

Comparative terms—alike, different, same, same as, different from, almost alike, others.

Figures of speech—as big as a ______, smaller than a ______, looks like a ______, others.

Position—here, there, beside, beneath, above, below, near, far, next to, over, under, with, inside, outside, others.

Sequence—after, before, at the same time, first, second, third, others.

This is by no means a complete list, but will serve as a sample. The development of language takes place at a rapid rate during kindergarten, and in formal and informal classroom activities. Talking with others gives children practice, and you can enjoy sharing descriptions and observations with your child in your activities on a daily basis. In kindergarten, children are encouraged to use sentences, and to express feelings, observations, comparisons, and interpretations. Language is listed first here, because it is basic to many other skill areas, and you can see clearly how vocabulary and expression in language provide readiness for reading, mathematics, social studies, and other areas.

Reading Readiness Skills

1. Spatial orientation—visual readiness in identifying an object in pictures, moving objects on a ground, tracing, making shapes, matching shapes in two areas, others.

2. Progression—top to bottom progressions, right to left progressions, sequencing of simple shapes, letter shapes, numbers.

3. Shape recognition—letter-symbol recognition, word recognition of own name, others.

4. Sound-symbol recognition—simple phonemes such as own names, one-syllable words, others.

5. Reading interest—story telling, listening to read-aloud stories, identifying pictures of story characters, characters' names, labels, others.

Mathematics

1. Counting—one to ten, possibly one to a hundred as appropriate individually. Use of counting games, matching numbers of objects in games. Recognizing numbers and numerals.

2. Categorization and classification—sort by differences and similarities, match by differences and similarities.

3. Shapes—recognize, describe, name, compare.

4. Groups and sets—compare, match, join, separate.

5. Patterns—identify, match, extend.

6. Measurement—use common measuring tools such as cup, quart, bucket, foot ruler, yard stick, string, "growth ladder," tape measure, and for time, clocks, 3-minute timer, others.

7. Money—identify change and paper money, make up change for small amounts such as 10¢, 25¢, one dollar.

Social Studies

1. Self concept—describe likenesses and differences with others, relationships, feelings, beliefs.

2. Family—family members, likenesses and differences in families, relationships.

3. School and friends—observe and describe groups, relationships, structures, changes.

4. Community—share observations and descriptions of community and community services, housing, stores, fire and police protection, medical services, water and utilities, others.

5. Environmental—share in activities to conserve water, energy, keep from littering, observe natural life in animals and plants, simple relationships of ecology.

6. Culture—gain awareness of other cultures, share descriptions of holidays, household customs, songs and art, others.

7. Career and work concepts—recognize and describe common jobs in the community, express interests and knowledge of work and play games involving role plays, costumes, and tools.

8. Emotions and relationships—share in activities, observe and describe feelings, observe simple causes and effects, find solutions to problems, plan activities and simple games with a partner and in small groups.

9. Economic principles—understand that wants and needs are unlimited; resources are limited, and that choices must be made. Simple concepts of basic

helter, education, health
l structure, and use of
eeds.

Science

1. Health and safety
2. Personal hygiene
3. Nutrition
4. Weather and seasons
5. Plants and animals
6. Minerals
7. Use of basic scientific vocabulary of observations and comparison
8. Use of simple scientific tools, for stirring, mixing, preserving, measuring, magnifying, etc.